Recent Advances in the Pathogenesis of Gastrointestinal Bacterial Infections

John Libbey Eurotext
127, avenue de la République
92120 Montrouge
Tél. : 01 46 73 06 60

John Libbey and Company Ltd
13, Smiths Yard, Summerley Street
London SW18 4HR, England
Tel. : 1 947 27 77

John Libbey CIC
Via L. Spallanzani, 11
00161, Rome, Italie
Tel. : 06 862 289

ISBN : 2-7420-0221-9

Recent Advances in the Pathogenesis of Gastrointestinal Bacterial Infections

Edited by
P. Rampal
P. Boquet

Postgraduate Course 1998
Nice, July 2-3

John Libbey EUROTEXT

The publication of this book was made possible
thanks to the support from the BIOCODEX Laboratories

Contents

Bacterial toxins in the gastrointestinal tract

List of contributors

Boquet P., INSERM U 452, Faculté de Médecine de Nice, 28, avenue de Valombrose, 06107 Nice Cedex 2, France.

Connell H., Department of Medical Microbiology, Lund University, Lund, Sweden.

Cornelis G., Microbial Pathogenesis Unit, Christian de Duve Institute of Cellular Pathology and Université Catholique de Louvain, UCL 74-49, B-1200 Brussels, Belgium.

Corthésy-Theulaz I., Department of Internal Medicine, Division of Gastroenterology, Centre Hospitalier Universitaire Vaudois, CH 1011 Lausanne, Switzerland.

Cossart P., Unité des Interactions Bactéries-Cellules, Institut Pasteur, 28, rue du Docteur-Roux, 75724 Paris Cedex 15, France.

Czerkinsky C., INSERM U 364, Faculté de Médecine, 28, avenue de Valombrose, 06107 Nice Cedex 2, France and Department of Medical Microbiology and Immunology, Göteborg University, Sweden.

Czerucka D., Laboratoire de Gastroentérologie, Faculté de Médecine, 28, avenue de Valombrose, 06107 Nice Cedex 2, France.

Debard N., Swiss Institute of Experimental Cancer Research and Institute of Biochemistry, University of Lausanne, CH-1066, Epalinges, Switzerland.

Fabbri A., Department of Ultrastructures, Istituto Superiore di Sanità, Viale Regina Elena 299, 00161 Rome, Italy.

Falzano L., Department of Ultrastructures, Istituto Superiore di Sanità, Viale Regina Elena 299, 00161 Rome, Italy.

Farthing M.J.G., Digestive Diseases Centre, St Bartholomew's and the Royal London School of Medicine and Dentistry, Turner Street, London, UK.

Fiorentini C., Department of Ultrastructures, Istituto Superiore di Sanità, Viale Regina Elena 299, 00161 Rome, Italy.

Frendéus B., Department of Medical Microbiology, Lund University, Lund, Sweden.

Ghiara P., Antica Farmacia Parenti, via Banchi di Sopra, 53100 Siena, Italy.

Godaly G., Department of Medical Microbiology, Lund University, Lund, Sweden.

Hang L., Department of Medical Microbiology, Lund University, Lund, Sweden.

Haraoka M., Department of Medical Microbiology, Lund University, Lund, Sweden.

Hathaway L., Swiss Institute of Experimental Cancer Research and Institute of Biochemistry, University of Lausanne, CH-1066, Epalinges, Switzerland.

Hedlund M., Department of Medical Microbiology, Lund University, Lund, Sweden.

Hirst T.R., Department of Pathology and Microbiology, School of Medical Sciences, University of Bristol, Bristol BS8 1TD, UK.

Just I., Institut für Pharmakologie und Toxikologie der Albert-Ludwigs-Universität Freiburg, Hermann-Herder-Street 5, D-79104 Freiburg, Germany.

Kraehenbuhl J.P., Swiss Institute for Experimental Cancer Research and Institute of Biochemistry, University of Lausanne, CH-1066, Epalinges, Switzerland.

Mestecky J., Departments of Microbiology and Medicine, University of Alabama at Birmingham, Birmingham, AL, USA.

Millar D.G., Department of Pathology and Microbiology, School of Medical Sciences, University of Bristol, Bristol BS8, 1TD, UK.

Nashar T.O., Department of Pathology and Microbiology, School of Medical Sciences, University of Bristol, Bristol BS8 1TD, UK.

Olsnes S., Institute for Cancer Research, The Norwegian Radium Hospital, Montebello, 031 Oslo, Norway.

Otto G., Department of Infectious Diseases, Lund University, Lund, Sweden.

Rampal P., Service de Gastroentérologie, Hôpital de l'Archet, Centre Hospitalier Universitaire et Faculté de Médecine, 28, avenue de Valombrose, 06107 Nice Cedex 2, France.

Rappuoli R., IRIS, Chiron SpA, via Fiorentina 1, 53100 Siena, Italy.

Sansonetti P., Unité de Pathogénie Microbienne Moléculaire, INSERM U 389, Institut Pasteur, 28, rue du Docteur-Roux, 75724 Paris Cedex 15, France.

Svanborg C., Department of Medical Microbiology, Lund University, Lund, Sweden.

Svensson M., Department of Medical Microbiology, Lund University, Lund, Sweden.

Tran Van Nhieu G., Unité de Pathogénie Microbienne Moléculaire, INSERM U 389, Institut Pasteur, 28, rue du Docteur-Roux, 75724 Paris Cedex 15, France.

Williams N.A., Department of Pathology and Microbiology, School of Medical Sciences, University of Bristol, Bristol BS8, 1TD, UK.

Wullr B., Department of Urology, Lund University, Lund, Sweden.

Foreword

According to a well-established practice in recent years, one of the regional EAGE Post-Graduate Courses is held in France, usually in early July. On behalf of the Governing Board of the Society, I am especially grateful to Patrick Rampal and Patrice Boquet for having proposed a superb programme of education on "Recent Advances in the Pathogenesis of Gastrointestinal Bacterial Infections" in Nice this year (July 2-3, 1998). The choice of this topic seems extremely relevant as the gastroenterologist in the late 90's is faced more and often with many diagnostic and therapeutic issues related to various bacteria that may affect one or several segments of the gastrointestinal tract. This holds true, not only for Third World countries, but also for our modern "advanced" societies. Since considerable progress has been made recently in our understanding of the pathogenesis of bacterial gastrointestinal infections, it seemed to be an appropriate time to bring together scientists and clinicians for a critical review of the different, frequently disappointing aspects of these challenging disorders. In addition to the virulence factors of the bacteria themselves, the pathophysiological mechanisms of bacterial infection involve many gut functions, *e.g.* local immune response, the action of toxins on intestinal secretions, and interactions with the enteric nervous system as well as effects on intestinal differentiation and apoptosis. All these mechanisms have been extensively described and discussed by the outstanding scientific experts of the International Faculty who accepted to contribute to this Course. It is noteworthy that interest in the several mechanisms reviewed here goes far beyond the specific field of infection. In fact they may actually provide decisive clues for future therapeutic advances, for instance in the development of antidiarrheal drug therapy or vaccines.

Both the editors and the authors of this excellent monograph are to be complimented for producing an impressive but quite accessible amount of knowledge in so short a time. This monograph will certainly be an essential work for all gastroenterologists and internists interested in the field of gastrointestinal infection.

This foreword also gives me the opportunity to make the first announcement of the next French EAGE Post-Graduate Course, which will be organised in Paris (July 1999) by Pr M. Mignon and J.F. Colombel and be dedicated to neuroendocrine tumours of the gut and inflammatory bowel disease. We are therefore confident that such continuous efforts and the ambitious programme of Education in Europe and in France will be increasingly attractive to young (and even less young) gastroenterologists. Because we need your support to achieve all these goals, I strongly invite you to join the Society and enjoy all the advantages and privileges of membership.

J.P. Galmiche, MD, FRCP
President of EAGE

Recent advances in the pathogenesis of gastrointestinal bacterial infections.
P. Rampal, P. Boquet, eds. John Libbey Eurotext, Paris © 1998, pp. 3-9.

Introductory remarks

Patrick Rampal, Dorota Czerucka

Service de Gastroentérologie, Hôpital de l'Archet, Centre Hospitalier Universitaire et Faculté de Médecine, Nice, France

Our knowledge about infectious diarrheal disease has expanded exponentially over the past two decades. Advances have been made in numerous disciplines, and integration of epidemiologic, clinical and laboratory data has improved our understanding of this group of diseases. We therefore felt it interesting to organize an EAGE course on this topic in order to familiarize participants with recent advances in the field.

Mucosal surfaces represent the major interface between the host and the environment. The intestinal mucosa, which is continually exposed to nutrients, is also in constant contact with microorganisms (viruses, bacteria, etc.). The gastrointestinal tract contains both nonpathogenic bacteria, which make up the normal intestinal flora, and transient bacteria that can colonize the GI tract and become pathogenic for the host. Colonization by gram-negative bacilli is the main cause of infection in human diseases.

Pathogenic bacteria differ from nonpathogenic bacteria by the expression of virulence factors. The genes coding for these factors are often grouped together in "blocks" referred to as pathogen islands, localized on either a plasmid or a chromosome [1]. These genes code for a variety of factors: (i) adhesins (lectin-like molecules that mediate bacterial adherence to the intestinal microvilli), (ii) invasins (bacterial proteins that mediate the invasion process, usually by subverting the cytoskeletal functions of the host epithelial cell), (iii) cytotoxins, delivered intra- or extracellularly, that cause epithelial cell death, and (iv) enterotoxins, which are usually secreted into the intestinal lumen and can modify ion exchange in enterocytes. Expression of one or more of these factors determines the mechanism(s) of pathogenesis. Acute bacterial diarrhea can be classified in two groups: toxigenic types, in which an enterotoxin is the major if not the sole pathogenic mechanism, and invasive forms, in which bacterial penetration of the mucosal surface is the primary event, but may be accompanied by production of an enterotoxin *(table I)*.

Table I. Classification of bacteria responsible for diarrhea as a function of their mechanism of pathogenicity

Pathogenicity factor	**Pathogen**	**Disease**	**Mechanism of pathogenicity**
Adhesion and cytotonicity	*V. cholerae*	Watery diarrhea	Cholera toxin (CT)
	Enterotoxigenic *E. coli* (ETEC)	Acute diarrhea; incriminated in travellers' diarrhea	LT (I and II) and ST (a and b) toxins
Adhesion and cytotoxicity	*Clostridium difficile*	Pseudomembranous enterocolitis	Toxins A and B
	Enteropathogenic *E. coli* (EPEC)	Acute diarrhea in children	Elimination of the microvilli and loosening of the tight junctions
	Enterohemorrhagic *E. coli* (EHEC)	Hemorrhagic colitis responsible for epidemics of food poisoning, associated with the hemolytic-uremic syndrome	Synthesis of Shiga-like toxin (SLT1 and SLT2), structural alteration
	Cell invasion	*Shigella*	Bacillary dysentery Penetration, multiplication, and invasion of adjacent cells
	Yersinia enterolitica, Yersinia pseudo-tuberculosis	Gastroenteritis	Penetration and dissemination towards other organs

Bacterial toxins in the GI tract

Toxins are one of numerous virulence factors involved in the pathogenesis of certain bacteria that do not invade the intestinal epithelium, such as *Vibrio cholerae*, *Escherichia coli* (ETEC), and *Clostridium difficile*. Their mechanism of action allow to distinguish the toxins that affect cell viability (cytotoxins) and those that affect regulation of ion transport in enterocytes (enterotoxins) (for review see [2]). Enterotoxigenic diarrhea is characterized by its watery nature, a relatively high sodium and chloride content, and the absence of morphological damage to the intestinal epithelium. The most widely studied enterotoxin is cholera toxin (CT), which is synthesized by *Vibrio cholerae*. CT presents homology with toxins produced by certain *E. coli*. Enterotoxigenic *E. coli* (ETEC) synthesizes both heat-labile (LT-1 and LT-II) and heat-stable (STa and STb) enterotoxins. LT-1 shares 80% sequence identity with CT: these toxins bind to the GM1 ganglioside receptor present on the apical membrane of enterocytes. LT-II toxin shares only 55% identity with CT, and recognizes a receptor different from GM1. All of these ADP-ribosylating toxins activate the enzyme adenylate cyclase, and this results in an increase in intracellular cyclic AMP. ST toxins are low molecular weight, heat-stable peptides that recognize an apically-located receptor: guanylate cyclase. ST toxins, which are also ADP-ribosylating toxins, activate guanylate cyclase, which leads to an increase in intracellular cGMP. cAMP and cGMP both activate cyclic nucleotide-dependent protein kinases, which results in phosphorylation and opening of the apical membrane chloride channel of crypt cells. cAMP also inhibits the action of the sodium/hydrogen exchanger and its associated anion exchanger in intestinal villi: this leads to a reduction in neutral sodium and chloride absorption by these cells. Neuronal pathways have been implicated in alteration of intestinal ion and fluid transport by CT, LT, STb and *Clostriium difficile (C. difficile)* toxin A. The exact mechanism of action of these toxins on the nerve pathway remains unclear. There is evidence that CT and STb may release serotonin (5-HT) from enterochromaffin cells; 5-HT might then activate the neuronal pathway *via* 5-HT_2, 5-HT_3 and 5-HT_4 neuronal receptors. However, serotonin secretion has not been observed in the presence of LT toxins. In the case of *C. difficile* toxin A, substances released by enterocytes undergoing necrosis might activate substance P-secreting neurons.

Cytotoxins affect epithelial cell viability by various mechanisms. Apoptosis, which occurs throught the activation of cell intrinsic suicide program, plays an important role in bacterial GI tract infections [3]. Activation of the apoptosis of macrophages and polymorphonuclear cells (PMNs) permits bacteria *(Shigella, Yersinia, Listeria monocytogenesis)* to neutralize the host immune defense system. Destruction of epithelial cells by apoptosis favors bacterial colonization and dissemination throughout the GI tract. Certain bacterial enterotoxins can affect regulation of apoptosis in epithelial cells. As shown by Fiorentini *et al.* [4, 5], *C. difficile* toxins A and B can induce apoptosis in IEC 6 cells. Inactivation of small GTP binding proteins (Rho, Rac, and Cdc24) by glucosylation appears to be the molecular mechanism by which *C. difficile* toxins mediate cytotoxic effects in cells. The resultant alteration in actin architecture leads to cell rounding and loss of adherence. Detached epithelial cells can produce cytokins (IL-8) capable of mediating inflammatory processes. The role of these phenomena in the pathogenesis of *C. difficile in vivo* remains to be demonstrated.

Inhibition of host cell apoptosis is another strategy used by bacteria to survive inside mammalian cells. One good example is cytotoxic necrotizing factor (CNF1), a cytotoxin synthesized by certain *E. coli*. After internalization into cells by endocytosis, CNF1 activates the Rho protein by deamination of the p21 Rho glutamin 63, which results in mutation into glutamic acid. The subsequent modification of cytoskeletal architecture gives epithelial cells a nonspecific phagocytic-like behavior that allows noninvasive bacteria to multiply and be transcytosed through the epithelium into the bloodstream. Strictly correlated with this finding is the fact that CNF1 can protect cells against apoptosis induced by ultraviolet radiation [6]. Recent studies suggest that CNF1 may modulate (probably through Rho activation) the expression of certain Bcl-$_2$ proteins implicated in the regulation of apoptosis. Shiga toxins (SLT1 and SLT2), identified in *Shigella dysenteriae* 1, are the putative cause of the much higher lethality of infections associated with this bacteria compared to other species of *Shigella* (for review see [7]). The endothelium is the primary target of these toxins that have enterotoxic, cytotoxic, and neurotoxic activities. SLT1 and SLT2 consist of two subunits [8]. The B-subunit recognizes the functional receptor, a globotraosyl ceramide (Gb_3). The A subunit consists of two fragments: A1 and A2. The N-glycosidase activity of SLT is located on the A1 fragment. These toxins block protein synthesis by hydrolyzing the adenine residue in position 4324 of the 28S ribosomal RNA [9]. Identical or similar toxins, called Shiga-like toxins or verotoxins, have been identified in enterohemorrhagic strains of *E. coli* (EHEC) associated with the hemolytic-uremic syndrome (HUS) [10]. Owing to the widespread involvement of Shiga and Shiga-like toxins in severe pathologies in both industrial and developing countries, considerable efforts are being made to develop vaccines against toxignic bacteria and toxins.

Invasive bacteria in the GI tract

Some bacteria affect the host by invading the intestinal epithelium. Toxigenic organisms characteristically involve the upper intestine, whereas invasive pathogens have a predilection for the lower bowel, and especially the distal ileum and the colon. The main histologic feature is mucosal ulceration with an acute inflammatory reaction in the *lamina propria*. The principal pathogens in this group are *Salmonella*, *Shigella*, invasive *E. coli* (EHEC), *Campylobacter*, and *Yersinia (table I)*. Despite important differences among these microorganisms, they all have a common property: mucosal invasion is the initial event in pathogenesis.

Formed of polarized cells linked together by tight junctions, the intestinal epithelium is an effective barrier against bacterial invasion. Certain pathogenic bacteria thus use the M cells present in the lymphoid structures of the epithelium (Peyer's patches) as a path through the mucosal barrier, resulting in local or systemic infections [11]. M cells are polarized epithelial cells connected to adjacent cells by tight junctions. Their apical membrane presents sparse microvilli covered by a thin layer of glycocalyx that facilitates bacterial adhesion. The apical membrane of M cells is thus more accessible to bacteria than enterocytes. The basolateral membrane of M cells is invaginated, forming an intracellular pocket into and out of which lymphocytes and macrophages migrate. M cells ensure nonselective internalization of antigens (molecules, particles and microorganisms) and their transport to cells in the central pocket. Numerous enteropathogens attach to M cells. Some, like enteroadherent *E. coli*, resist internalization by M cells. Others, such as *Vibrio cholerae*, are transported by M cells but are then phagocytosed and degraded by macrophages. Finally, a certain number of invasive pathogens (for example *Shigella*, *Salmonella*, and *Yersinia*) preferentially use M cells as a means to penetrate the intestinal barrier and escape the host immune system.

Shigella are foodborne pathogens responsible for acute intestinal infections in humans. Clinical manifestations range from mild, watery diarrhea to dysentery (severe diarrhea with blood and mucus in the stools). The two main species responsible for severe dysentery are *Shigella flexeneri* and *Shigella dysenteriae* serotype 1. A crucial step in bacillary dysentery due to *Shigella flexenerei* is bacterial invasion of the colon mucosa (for review see [12, 13, 14]). After penetrating the intestinal barrier, essentially by M cells, *Shigella* penetrates the macrophage, induces apoptosis, then spreads to adjacent enterocytes by the basolateral membrane, thereby escaping destruction by lymphocytes [3]. The ability of *Shigella* to enter epithelial cells is determined by a 31 kB region on the virulence plasmid. This region contains up to

30 different genes, almost all of which have been studied by directed mutagenesis. Some, like Invasion Plasmid Antigens: Ipa B, C, D are directly implicated in the entry process; Ipa B and D may also play a role in regulation of secretion while Ipa A appears to optimize entry efficiency [15]. *Shigella* is characterized by its actin-based motility in cells. The icsA gene on the virulence plasmid of *S. flexenerei* is central to this intracellular motility. This gene codes for a 120 kD protein that appears implicated in actin polymerization, which is required for motility along the actin filaments.

Listeria monocytogenesis is another example of a bacteria capable of moving from one cell to another. This foodborne pathogen, which causes meningitis, menigo-encepalitis and gastroenteritis in humans, is unique in its capability to cross three barriers during infection: the intestinal barrier, the brain-blood barrier, and/or the placental barrier. Recent data indicate that *L. monocytogenesis* crosses the intestinal barrier through enterocytes or M cells [16]. The bacteria survive and even replicate in macrophages, then reach other organs such as the liver or spleen by hematogenous or lymphatic spread. Entry into mammalian cells is mediated by at least two bacterial factors: internalin InlA and InlB (for review see [17]). The internalin receptor has been identified: this adhesion molecule, E-cadherin, is mainly expressed at the adherens junction and on the basolateral surface of enterocytes. Internalin is sufficient to promote bacterial entry into the cell. InlB is found on both the surface of the bacteria and in the bacterial supernatant. This protein has similarities with internalin but its receptor has not been identified. This motility of *L. monocytogenesis*, which depends on actin polymerization, is initiated by the protein ActA present on the bacterial membrane.

Numerous *Yersinia* species are pathogenic for humans and rodents: *Y. pestis* is implicated in bubonic plague, *Y. pseudotuberculosis* causes adenitis and septicemia, and *Y. enterocolitica* causes a broad range of gastrointestinal syndromes in humans. The 70 kB plasmid PYV, which encodes the Yops proteins, enables *Yersinia* to survive and multiply in the host lymphoid tissues. This integrated system permits the synthesis and release of proteins into the host cytosol. This system is composed of four elements: (i) a type III secretion system called Ysc that allows secretion of Yops proteins; (ii) the YopB, YopD, LerD and LerV gene system that allows delivery of bacterial protein into the host cytosol; (iii) control elements (YopN and TyeA); and (iv) a set of effector proteins (YopE, YopH, YopM, YpkA/YopO, YopP/YopJ, YopT) that alter the function of the host cell (for review see [18]).

Vaccines production as new therapeutic strategy

The mucosa are exposed to multiple bacterial and viral antigens. The gastric and intestinal mucosa which are also exposed to nutrient antigens, constitute a barrier against these antigens and have a specialized compartmentalized immune system called Gut-Associated Lymphoid Structure (GALT) (for review see [19]). The GALT consists of Peyer's patches and the solitary follicles present in the intestinal mucosa. It has three main function: to protect against colonization and invasion by dangerous microbes, to prevent uptake of undegraded antigens (food proteins for exemple) and to prevent development of potentially harmfull immune responses to these antigens. The mucosa secrete immunoglobulins in response to antigens: immunoglobulin A (IgA), the predominant type in the intestinal mucosa, is produced essentially by activated B lymphocytes present in the follicles and the plasmocytes of the *lamina propria* (for review see [20]). SIgA antibodies provide "immune exclusion" of bacterial and viral pathogens, bacterial toxins and other potentially harmful molecules. It is now well established that in order to be efficacious, vaccines against mucosal infectious must stimulate the mucosal immune system, and that this goal is usually better achieved by administrating immunogens by the oral route rather than parenterally. The feeding of an antigen prior to parental immunization can induce systemic unresponsiveness or "oral tolerance" instead of immunity. The factors determining wheteher immunity or tolerance results from antigens encounter in the gut are not well understood, but presumably the answer lies in complexe regulatory cell interactions within the GALT. It has been also assumed that only live vaccines would efficiently stimulate a mucosal immune response. The use of live attenuated recombinant bacteria and viruses, which can be genetically engineered to express unrelated antigens are currently under investigation. However, with the main bacterial vector candidates tested, foreign antiges are not always expressed in sufficient quantities. To promote mucosal and systemic antibody responses, CT, the most potent mucosal immunogen and adjuvant known so far and its analog *E. coli* LT enterotoxin where co-administrated with either unconjugated or conjugated antigens. I.C. Theulaz will expose the problems associated with the choose of reliable immunological markers and the importance of mucosal adjuvant in the vaccination against *Helicobacter pylori*. Moreover, GALT is in contact with the immune system associated with other mucosal systems such as the respiratory tract (Bronchial Associated Lymphoid Tissue: BALT) and the urogenital tract: these systems constitute the Mucosal-Associated Lymphoid Tissues (MALT). The MALT lymphoid system is considered distinct from the systemic lymphoid organs. One reason for this distinction is the fact that the lymphoid cells of this system circulate throughout the mucosal areas. Antigenic stimulation of a mucosal membrane can thus induce an antibody response in another mucosal area. The concept of a common mucosal immune system open an attractive strategy to develop oral vaccines against for exemple infections of the buccal, ocular, respiratory, and genital mucosa.

Research on the genetic bases of bacterial pathogenesis is useful not only for comprehension of pathogenic phenomena and the evolution of species, but also contributes to the elaboration of new vaccines and the development of sensitive and specific diagnostic tools.

References

1. Groisman EA, Ochman H. Pathogenicity islands: bacterial evolution in quantum leaps. *Cell* 1996; 87: 791-4.
2. Sears CL, Kaper JB. Enteric bacterial toxins: mechanisms of action and linkage to intestinal secretion. *Microbial Rev* 1996; 60: 167-215.

3. Zychlinsky A, Sansonetti PJ. Apoptosis in bacterial pathogenesis. *J Clin Invest* 1997; 100: 493-6.
4. Fiorentini C, Donelli G, Nicotera P, Thelestam M. *Clostridium difficile* toxin A elicits Ca^{2+}-independent cytotoxic effects in cultured normal crypt cells. *Infect Immun* 1993; 61: 3988-93.
5. Fiorentini C, Fabbri A, Falzano L, Fattorossi A, Matarrese P, Rivabene R, Donelli G. *Clostridium difficile* toxin B induces apoptosis in intestinal cultured cells. *Infect Immun* 1998; in press.
6. Fiorentini C, Fabbri A, Matarrese P, Falzano L, Boquet P, Malorni W. Hinderance of apoptosis and phagocytic behaviour induced by *E. coli* necrozing factor 1 (CNF1): two related activities in epithelial cells. *Biochem Biophys Res Commun* 1997; 241: 341-6.
7. O'Brien AD, Holmes RK. Shiga and Shiga-like toxins. *Microbiol Rev* 1987; 51: 206-20.
8. Olnes S, Reisbig R, Eiklid K. Subunit structure of *Shigella* cytotoxin. *J Biol Chem* 1981; 256: 8723-38.
9. Endo Y, Tsurugi K, Yutsudo T, Takeda Y, Ogasawara T, Igarashi K. Site of action of a vero toxin (VT2) from *Escherichia coli* O157: H7 and Shiga toxin on eucaryotic ribosomes. RNA N-glycosidase activity of the toxins. *Eur J Biochem* 1988; 171: 45-50.
10. Kamali MA, Steele BT, Petric M, Lim C. Sporadic cases of haemolytic-uraemic syndrome associated with faecal cytotoxin and cytotoxin-producing *Escherichia coli* in stools. *Lancet* 1983; 1: 619-20.
11. Siebers A, Finlay BB. M cells and the pathogenesis of mucosal and systemic infections. *Trends Microbiol* 1996; 4: 22-9.
12. Ménard R, Dehio C, Sansonetti PJ. Bacterial entry into epithelial cells: the paradigm of Shigella. *Trends Microbiol* 1996; 4: 220-6.
13. Parsot CR, Sansonetti PJ. Invasion and pathogenesis of Shigella infections. *Curr Top Microbiol Immunol* 1996; 209: 25-42.
14. Sansonetti PJ. Molecular mechanisms of cell and tissue invasion by *Shigella flexeneri. Infect Agents Dis* 1993; 2: 201-6.
15. Tran Van Nhieu G, Ben Zeev A, Sansonetti PJ. Modulation of bacterial entry into epithelial cells by interaction between vinculin and the *Shigella* IpaA invasin. *EMBO J* 1997; 16: 2717-29.
16. Pron B, Boumaila C, Jaubert F, Sarnacki S, Monnet JP, Gaillard JL. Comprehensive study of the intestinal stage of listeriosis in rat ligated ileal loop system. *Infect Immun* 1998; 66, 747-55.
17. Irekon K, Cossart P. Host-pathogen interactions during entry and actin-based movement of *Listeria monocytogenesis. Annu Rev Genet* 1997; 31: 113-38.
18. Cornelis GR, Wolf-Watz H. The *Yersinia* Yop virulon: a bacterial system for subverting enkaryotic cells. *Mol Microbiol* 1997; 23: 861-7.
19. Brandzaeg P. Basic of mucosal immunity: a major adaptive defence system. *The immunologist* 1995; 3: 89-95.
20. Czerkinsky C, Holmgren J. The mucosal immune system and prospects for anti-infectious and anti-inflammatory vaccines. *The immunologist* 1995; 3: 97-103.
21. Parsot C. *Shigella flexeneri*: genetics of entry and intercellular dissemination in epithelial cells. In: Dangl JL, ed. *Bacterial pathogenesis of plants and animal, molecular and cellular mechanisms*. Springer Verlag, 1994: 217-41.

Helicobacter pylori

Recent advances in the pathogenesis of gastrointestinal bacterial infections.
P. Rampal, P. Boquet, eds. John Libbey Eurotext, Paris © 1998, pp. 13-23.

Virulence factors of *Helicobacter pylori*

Rino Rappuoli, Paolo Ghiara

IRIS, Chiron SpA, Via Fiorentina 1, 53100 Siena, Italy

Helicobacter pylori is a spiral, gram negative microaerophilic bacterium that colonizes the human stomach. Infection with this bacterium occurs early in life and persists life-long. Approximately two-thirds of the human population is infected by *H. pylori*. The frequency of infection depends on the age and the socio-economical status. In developing countries up to 80% of the population is infected by the age of ten. In developed countries, infection is approximately 10% at ten years and 40-50% in 50-year olds. Stomach colonization by *H. pylori* is associated with chronic gastritis, peptic ulcer, gastric adenocarcinoma and MALT lymphoma [1-3]. Gastritis is present at different degrees in all infected people and at any time develops into symptomatic diseases in only about 10% of them.

Peptic ulcers, MALT lymphoma and gastric adenocarcinoma develop following years and often decades of chronic infection and for this reason *H. pylori* has been called a "slow bacterium". Eradication is achieved with a combination of antibiotics (*i.e.* clarithromycin, amoxycillin, metronidazole) plus antisecretory drugs (*i.e.* omeprazole), but the increasing occurrence of antibiotic resistance is dampening the efficacy of such therapies.

During the last five years information has increased exponentially about the molecular pathogenesis of the infection and the entire *H. pylori* genome has been described. Clinical isolates of *H. pylori* can be divided into more virulent, or Type I, and less virulent, or Type II [4]. Type II are poor pathogens and are associated only with a mild gastritis. Type I are virulent and are associated with all the severe consequences of the infection including severe gastritis, peptic ulcer, MALT lymphoma and gastric cancer [5-7].

Much effort is being employed to the characterization of relevant virulence factors also with the aim of identifying putative candidates for vaccine formulations.

The more virulent Type I strains harbour a "pathogenicity island"

A major difference between Type I and Type II bacteria resides in a 40 kilobase pair of DNA (cag locus), that is present in Type I bacteria only and that is named pathogenicity island (PAI) [8]. This DNA locus has been acquired during evolution from an unknown organism and has provided *H. pylori* with an increased virulence. The PAI codes for approximately 30 genes, most of which are predicted to code for membrane-associated proteins. Five of these proteins are homologous to components of Type IV secretory machines found in *Agobacterium tumefaciens*, *Bordetella pertussis*, and *Escherichia coli*, suggesting that the PAI may also encode a secretion machinery. As yet it is not known which are the components that are secreted by the cag PAI, however, it is well established that the cag PAI plays a crucial role in virulence because in addition to the correlates with disease discussed above, the presence of the PAI is essential *in vitro* for a number of contact-dependent activities in co-cultured eukaryotic cells such as: i) induction of the pro-inflammatory lymphokine IL-8; ii) tyrosine phosphorylation of a 145 kDa protein; iii) pedestal formation; iv) NF-kB activation. Inactivation of most of the genes coded by the cag PAI abolishes all the above activities [8, 9].

The cag PAI codes also for an immunodominant protein with unknown function, that is not necessary for cag function. This protein was the first one to be discovered in Type I bacteria and the cag PAI derived its name from it. CagA is variable in size from 120 to 160 kDa and the variability is due to the presence of one or more repeats of a 100 base pairs fragment of the gene. Being CagA very immunogenic, antibodies to this protein in Western countries have been shown to correlate with infection with Type I bacteria and severe disease. In Eastern countries (China, Japan) where people are infected almost entirely by Type I bacteria, the diagnostic value of this protein is less relevant.

Type I bacteria are able to exert direct cytotoxicity to gastric epithelial cells

H. pylori Type I strains produce a secreted cytotoxin that induces cytoplasmic vacuolation in eukaryotic cells and epithelial erosion when administered orally to mice [10]. Biological and structural data suggest similarities to the AB family of dichain toxins which are formed of an enzymatically active moiety (A) and a receptor binding and translocation moiety (B). VacA is produced as a 140 kDa precursor which is cleaved at the C-terminal domain and released into the extracellular milieu as a 95 kDa mature protein that assembles into large oligomeric structures with hexameric or heptameric radial symmetry [11, 12]. Each monomer can be proteolytically cleaved at a specific site into two fragments of 37 kDa and 58 kDa that remain associated after cleavage, suggesting that they may represent two distinct cytotoxin subunits [13].

It has been recently shown that the cytotoxin is able to bind to and to be internalized by the target cell [14], and a potential receptor has been identified as a membrane associated protein of 140 kDa [15, 16]. Intracellular expression of a transfected *vacA* gene results in cell vacuolation indicating activity of the toxin in the cytoplasm [17]. The toxicity is due to a specific block of fluid phase endocytosis that induces the accumulation of a post-endosomal compartment [18, 19]. Moreover, VacA interfers with antigen presentation by B-cells by impairing processing and maturation of antigen by the antigen presenting cell [20].

Only approximately 50% of clinical isolates of *H. pylori* produce cytotoxic activity in a HeLa cell vacuolation assay. However, most isolates (80%) have a functionally expressed *vacA* gene. Toxicity has been associated with mosaicism in *vacA* genes in toxic and non-toxic isolates [21]. Three different signal-peptide sequences (s1a, s1b and s2) and two variants of the mode-region (m1 and m2) have been described. Isolates with the s1-m1 forms are toxic, while the s2-m2 forms are essentially non toxic. The M region spans approximately 300 aminoacids at the carboxy-terminus of the P58 subunit. However, while *in vitro* toxicity on HeLa cells is only associated with the s1-m1 allele, to date there is no evidence showing that the m2 allele is associated with milder forms of the disease. On the contrary, the m2 allele has been found associated with peptic ulcer [22] and is prevalent in the population where peptic ulcer and gastric cancer have also a high incidence.

Recent data show that also the m2 toxin is toxic when added to other cell types such as primary culture human gastric cells or a different epithelial cell line such as RK-13 (Reyrat *et al.*, manuscript submitted).

Urease

Urease is a nickel-dependent enzyme that catalyzes the hydrolysis of urea to form ammonia and carbon dioxide. The protein is produced in large amounts intracellularly (about 6% of water extractable proteins) and is released extracellularly upon cell lysis. The enzyme is essential for colonization possibly because it efficiently provides large amounts of ammonia, which is an important source of nitrogen for the metabolism and, together with CO_2, it is also hypothesized to form a cloud of neutral pH which protects the bacterium form the acid environment of the stomach.

The native enzyme is composed of two subunits, UreA (27 kDa) and ureB (62 kDa), that are stably associated in a 1:1 heterodimer. The heterodimers are then assembled together to form a macromolecular $(A{:}B)_6$ ring-like structure of high molecular mass [23, 24]. The two urease subunits are encoded by ureA and ureB genes, that belong to a large operon composed of nine genes (named A through I) [25].

Urease has been reported to have pro-inflammatory activities *in vitro* and it is present in deep mucosal tissue (lamina propria), whereas *H. pylori* cells are absent [26, 27]. However, a recent study that employed a mouse model of acute gastric injury failed to sustain this hypothesis [28].

Urease has been reported by many groups to be a protective antigen in animal models of infection [29].

Flagellins

H. pylori bears 4-6 sheathed polar flagella. These flagella are constituted by a basal portion, that contains the motor and the hook structure, and a central filament that is enveloped in a sheath composed of a bi-layered membrane with a composition closely resembling that of the outer membrane of the cell wall. Motility is essential for gastric colonization by *H. pylori*, thus it is considered a major virulence factor. The flagellin filament is composed by a major 53 kDa flagellin molecule (FlaA). Sequence alignments with other flagellin genes demonstrates an high degree of homology (about 60%) at the C- and N-termini with the related genus *Campylobacter*, while the central domain of the molecule is much less conserved. Further investigations have shown the presence of a second flagellin molecule with a slightly higher molecular mass (54 kDa). This second flagellin has been named FlaB. Targeted disruption of *flaA* gene results in complete loss of flagellum, while the *flaB* mutants are less motile but flagellated [30]. In a more recent study, in which *flaAflaB* double mutants were also used, FlaB expression was shown to be essential for optimal motility of *H. pylori* [31]. The reasons for flagellin gene duplication in *H. pylori* is unclear, however, similar duplications of flagellin genes occur in other gastrointestinal pathogens and may represent a functional advantage.

Heat shock proteins

Two *H. pylori* proteins, named HspA and HspB, that are functionally equivalent to *E. coli* GroES and GroEL, respectively, are encoded by a bi-cistronic operon [32, 33]. The HspA protein bears at its C-terminus a cysteine- and histidine-rich stretch resembling a nickel-binding domain, which is absent from the other known GroES moleculars. Co-expression in *E. coli* of *hspB* gene with Urease gene cluster *(ureA-BEFGHI)* has shown a significant increase in the secretion of active urease enzyme, suggesting that also in *H. pylori* these kind of proteins may function as chaperonins [34].

Catalase and superoxide dismutase

H. pylori can be actively phagocytosed by macrophages and neutrophils. However, in the absence of opsonins, the bacterium is able to survive within the phagocyte. A major killing mechanism of phagocytes is represented by the activation of the oxidative burst that leads to the formation of hydrogen peroxide and highly reactive superoxide anions. To counteract this toxic activity *H. pylori*, like many other pathogens, has evolved to express a superoxide dismutase (SOD) that catalyzes the dismutation of superoxide anions and catalase, which neutralizes the hydrogen peroxide. Catalase has been recently reported as a protective antigen in the *H. pylori* mouse model (see below) [35].

Adhesins

H. pylori cells are usually found swimmming in the mucous gel lining the gastric mucosa. A small percentage of bacteria can also tightly adhere to the luminl surface of gastric cells and in the spaces between adjacent cells. This clear-cut specificity indicates that adhesion is mediated by specific recognition between structures present on the bacterium and on the host gastric cells. Many putative adhesins have been characterized (reviewed in [36]) and active or passive immunization against these molecules could be relevant to prevent or combat the *H. pylori* infection.

Recent elegant studies by Boren *et al.* have shown that blood group O antigen Le^b, expressed by the human gastric mucosa, is also involved in *H. pylori* adhesion [37, 38]. These observations account for the known higher susceptibility of people carrying these antigens to develop peptic ulcer disease. The Le^b binding adhesin, BabA, has been recently identified and characterized, and the Le^b binding phenotype among the clinical isolates has been associated with the presence of the cag PAI [39].

Active immunization against structures like BabA involved in *H. pylori* adhesion to epithelial cells could be important to protect the host from colonization.

LPS

H. pylori lipopolysaccharide (LPS), like other Gram negative LPS, consists of a lipid component, Lipid A, that ensures incorporation into the outer layer of the outer membrane, and an outer carbohydrate domain that spans into the outer environment. Lipid A structure is quite conserved among different strains [40] and its biological activity has been reported to be low [41] as compared to *E. coli* LPS.

Of interest are recent data [42] indicating that the O side chain can mimic the structure of the blood group antigens Le^x and Le^y. These antigens are also expressed in the gastric mucosa. Thus this mimicry of gastric mucosa antigens by *H. pylori* LPS may play an important role in evading the immune response and may also represent a structural explanation of the finding [43], whereby they hypothesized the generation of autoantibodies reacting to the gastric mucosa upon chronic infection. Interesting is also a recent report that suggests that the LPS bearing these Le^x/Le^y-like structures appears to be more frequently expressed by Type I, more virulent, strains [44].

Steps towards the development of a vaccine

To define the protective immunity against *H. pylori* infection, and thus identify effective vaccination strategies, it is important to develop good animal models of infection that are relevant to the human disease.

Chen *et al.*, using the surrogate species *Helicobacter felis*, reported for the first time that vaccination against *Helicobacter* was feasible by immunizing the mice orally with bacterial lysates plus cholera toxin (CT) as mucosal adjuvant [45]. The *H. felis* model has, however, poor relevance to the human disease because a) it uses a bacterium that is not an human pathogen, b) *H. felis* is not able to express the pathogenic determinants (*i.e.* VacA and CagA) that have been demonstrated to be important in human pathology. Therefore, this model, although having been the first conveniently available model of infection with an *Helicobacter*, may not be ideal for giving insight into the pathogenesis of human infection and for the development of human vaccines.

Previous attempts to establish persistent infection in the normal mice had only poor success. Persistent infection could be obtained only by using nude or germ-free mice, whose peculiar immune systems limit their use to develop relevant vaccination systems (reviewed in [36]).

We have been able to obtain infections detectable for at least 12 weeks by using very fresh clinical isolates cultured in microaerophilic conditions for no more that three weeks after isolation from the patient's biopsies. Bacteria isolated from infected mice two weeks after the primary inoculum were then orally inoculated to other mice. Several cycles of isolation-reinoculation were then performed with an apparent increase in colonization efficiency. This suggests that "good colonizers" could be selected and maintained by passaging *in vivo* the bacteria. Using these "mouse-adapted" *H. pylori* strains we could obtain infections that persist for long time (> 12 months) with no signs of decrease.

Infections were performed with phenotypically characterized *H. pylori* strains. A mild gastritis was observed in all infected mice after 4-8 weeks, but in mice infected with Type I strains the gastric pathology was more evident and consisted of both gastritis and superficial erosions of epithelium [46]. Chronic infection induces the appearance of mucosal lyphoid aggregates (*i.e.* follicular gastritis) [47].

The availability of this new mouse model of *H.pylori* infection and disease has allowed to study the pathogenesis and to better assess the feasibility of vaccine in animal model that is highly relevant to human disease.

We have reported successful protection of mice from infection by *H. pylori* following intragastric immunization with *H. pylori* antigens together with the heat-labile enterotoxin of *E. coli* (LT) as mucosal adjuvant [46]. While immunization with urease or total bacterial lysates was able to protect mice from infection by both Type I and Type II strains, the VacA induced a Type I-specific protection. This indicated that the observed protection was due to antigen-specific immune mechanisms. The immune effector mechanism responsible in this mouse model of vaccination for the observed protection has not been identified. There is no correlation with protection and induction of secretory IgA (Ghiara, De Magistris and Di Tommaso, unpublished observations). Further studies are ongoing in order to define the correlate of protective immunity.

The mouse model of persistent infection has been further exploited to address two major issues: a) the identification of a non toxic mucosal adjuvant, and b) the identification of other *H. pylori* antigens as vaccine candidates.

The highly toxic activity of LT is a major drawback to its use as an adjuvant in humans. The adjuvant activity of this molecule, as the one of its homologous CT, has been linked to their strong ADP-ribosylating activity [51]. In spite of these published data, our group at Chiron SpA was able to obtain by site-directed mutagenesis a number of non-toxic and non-enzymatically active mutants of LT that retained a good adjuvant activity to antigens co-delivered at mucosal sites [52].

These non-toxic molecules have been therefore used as adjuvants in oral immunizations of mice. One of them, LTK63, was selected for its high stability to proteases [53] and was then used to assess the potential of *H. pylori* antigens as vaccine candidate in the mouse model.

A summary of the prophylactic oral vaccination data obtained so far in mouse models is reported in *Table I.*

Mucosal vaccination strategies can be exploited also for eradication of otherwise chronic infections. The first evidence of the feasibility of this therapeutic approach in the *Helicobacter* field was obtained by Doidge *et al.*, who showed that an established infection by *H. felis* in the mouse could be eradicated by therapeutic vaccination using whole cell sonicates and CT [54]. This result was then reproduced in the same animal model using recombinant urease as antigen [55]. Natural infection of ferrets by their natural gastric pathogen *Helicobacter mustelae* can be partially eradicated by intragastric therapeutic vaccination with recombinant urease holoenzyme [56].

Using the new mouse model of *H. pylori* infection in the mouse we have shown that a completely non toxic vaccine formulation consisting of LTK63 and the recombinant non toxic VacA (TOX100) could efficiently eradicate the infection [57].

Table I. Antigens tested in prophylactic vaccination in mouse models

Antigen	Adjuvant	Infection with	% protection	References
Sonicate	CT, LT, LTK63	*H. pylori*	80-100	[46, 47]
	CT	*H. felis*	70	[48]
Formalin killed bacteria	LTK63	*H. pylori*	100	[47]
Urease	LT, CT, LTK63	*H. pylori*	80	[46, 47]
	LT, CT	*H. felis*	70	[48]
UreB subunit	LT, CT	*H. felis*	25-70	[48, 49]
Heat shock proteins	CT	*H. felis*	70	[50]
Heat shock protein + UreB	LT	*H. felis*	100	[50]
Catalase	CT	*H. pylori*	80	[35]
VacA	LT, CT, LTK63	*H. pylori*	80	[46, 47]
CagA	LTK63	*H. pylori*	80	[47]

The current status of therapeutic vaccination data available in literature is summarized in *Table II*.

Table II. Current status of therapeutic vaccination studies in animal models

Infection with	Animal species	Antigen	Adjuvant	% eradication	Reference
H. pylori	mouse	sonicate	LTK63	70	[57]
		VacA	LTK63	90	[57]
H. felis	mouse	sonicate	CT	70	[54]
		UreB	CT	90	[55]
H. mustelae	ferret	Urease	CT	30	[56]

Concluding remarks

The studies on molecular pathogenesis of *H. pylori* are leading to a detailed description of several virulence factors that are responsible of the onset and maintenance of the disease. The mouse model of persistent *H. pylori* infection is a powerful tool to study the pathogenesis *in vivo* and for the preclinical tests of vaccine candidates. This new model has established the concept of the feasibility of vaccination against *H. pylori*. The next challenge will be to transfer the experience accumulated on the laboratory animals to clinical trials. A Phase I safety trial has recently been performed with recombinant urease [58]. Further clinical trials are planned that will assess the feasibility of human vaccination against this important pathogen.

References

1. Blaser MJ, Parsonnet J. Parasitism by the "slow'' bacterium *Helicobacter pylori* leads to altered gastric homeostasis and neoplasia. *J Clin Invest* 1994; 94: 4-8.
2. Parsonnet J, Friedman GD, Vandersteen DP, Chang Y, Vogelman JH, Orentreich N, Sibley RK. *Helicobacter pylori* infection and the risk of gastric carcinoma. *N Engl J Med* 1991; 325: 1127-31.
3. Parsonnet J, Hansen S, Rodriguez L, Gelb AB, Warnke RA, Jellum E, Orentreich N, Vogelman HJ, Friedman GD. *Helicobacter pylori* infection and gastric lymphoma. *N Engl J Med* 1994; 330: 1267-71.
4. Xiang Z, Censini S, Bayeli PF, Telford JL, Figura N, Rappuoli R, Covacci A. Analysis of expression of CagA and VacA virulence factors in 43 strains of *Helicobacter pylori* reveals that clinical isolates can be divided into two major types and that CagA is not necessary for expression of the vaculating cytotoxin. *Infect Immun* 1995; 63: 94-8.
5. Covacci A, Censini S, Bugnoli M, Petracca R, Burroni D, Macchia G, Massone A, Papini E, Xiang Z, Figura N, Rappuoli R. Molecular characterization of the 128-kDa immunodominant antigen of *Helicobacter pylori* associated with cytotoxicity and duodenal ulcer. *Proc Natl Acad Sci USA* 1993; 90: 5791-5.
6. Eck M, Schmausser B, Haas R, Greiner A, Czub S, Muller-Hermelink HK. MALT-type lymphoma of the stomach is associated with *Helicobacter pylori* strains expressing the CagA protein. *Gastroenterol* 1997; 112: 1482-6.

7. Blaser MJ, Perez-Perez GI, Kleanthous H, Cover TL, Peek RM, Chyou PH, Stemmermann GN, Nomura A. Infection with *Helicobacter pylori* strains possessing cagA is associated with an increased risk of developing adenocarcinoma of the stomach. *Cancer Res* 1995; 55: 2111-5.
8. Censini S, Lange C, Xiang ZY, Crabtree JE, Ghiara P, Borodovsky M, Rappuoli R, Covacci A. Cag, a pathogenicity island of *Helicobacter pylori*, encodes Type I-specific and disease-associated virulence factors. *Proc Natl Acad Sci USA* 1996; 93: 14648-53.
9. Covacci A, Falkow S, Berg DE, Rappuoli R. Did the inheritance of a pathogenicity island modify the virulence of *Helicobacter pylori*? *Trends Microbiol* 1997; 5: 205-8.
10. Telford JL, Covacci A, Ghiara P, Montecucco C, Rappuoli R. Unravelling the pathogenic role of *Helicobacter pylori* in peptic ulcer: potential for new therapies and vaccines. *Trends Biotechnol* 1994; 12: 420-6.
11. Lupetti P, Heuser JE, Manetti R, Massari P, Lanzavecchia S, Bellon PL, Dallai R, Rappuoli R, Telford JL. Oligomeric and subunit structure of the *Helicobacter pylori* vacuolating cytotoxin. *J Cell Biol* 1996; 133: 801-7.
12. Cover TL, Hanson PI, Heuser JE. Acid-induced dissociation of VacA, the *Helicobacter pylori* vacuolating cytotoxin, reveals its pattern of assembly. *J Cell Biol* 1997; 138: 759-69.
13. Telford JL, Ghiara P, Dell'Orco M, Comanducci M, Burroni D, Bugnoli M, Tecce MF, Censini S, Covacci A, Xiang ZY, Papini E, Montecucco C, Parente L, Rappuoli R. Gene structure of the *Helicobacter pylori* cytotoxin and evidence of its key role in gastric disease. *J Exp Med* 1994; 179: 1653-8.
14. Garner JA, Cover TL. Binding and internalization of the *Helicobacter pylori* vacuolating cytotoxin by epithelial. *Infect Immun* 1996; 64 (10): 4197-203.
15. Massari P, Manetti R, Burroni D, Nuti S, Norais N, Rappuoli R, Telford JL. Binding of the *Helicobacter pylori* vacuolating cytotoxin to target cells. *Infect Immun* (in press).
16. Yahiro K, Niidome T, Hatakeyma T, Aoyagi H, Kurazono H, Padilla PI, Wada A, Hirayama T. *Helicobacter pylori* vacuolating cytotoxin binds to the 140-kDa protein in human gastric cancer cell lines, AZ-521 and AGS. *Biochem Biophys Res Comm* 1997; 238: 62-9.
17. De Bernard M, Aricò B, Papini E, Rizzuto R, Grandi G, Rappuoli R, Montecucco C. *Helicobacter pylori* toxin VacA induces vacuole formation by acting in the cell cytosol. *Mol Microbiol* 1997; 26 (4): 665-74.
18. Papini E, Satin B, Bucci C, De Bernard M, Telford JL, Manetti R, Rappuoli R, Zerial M, Montecucco C. The small GTP-binding protein rab7 is essential for cellular vacuolation induced by *Helicobacter pylori* cytotoxin. *EMBO J* 1997; 16 (1): 15-24.
19. Papini E, De Bernard M, Milia E, Zerial M, Bugnoli M, Rappuoli R, Montecucco C. Cellular vacuoles induced by *Helicobacter pylori* originate from late endosomal compartments. *Proc Natl Acad Sci USA* 1994; 91 (21): 9720-4.
20. Molinari M, Salio M, Galli C, Norais N, Rappuoli R, Lanzavecchia A, Montecucco C. Selective inhibition of Ii-dependent antigen presentation by *Helicobacter pylori* toxin VacA. *J Exp Med* 1998; 187 (1): 135-40.
21. Atherton JC, Cao P, Peek RM, Tummuru MKR, Blaser MJ, Cover TL. Mosaicism in vacuolating cytotoxin alleles of *Helicobacter pylori* – association of specific vacA types with cytotoxin production and peptic ulceration. *J Biol Chem* 1995; 270: 17771-7.
22. Pagliaccia C, de Bernard M, Lupetti P, Xuhuai J, Burroni D, Cover TL, Papini E, Rappuoli R, Telford JL, Reyrat JM. The m2 of the *Helicobacter pylori* cytotoxin has cell type-specific vacuolating activity. Submitted.
23. Dunn BE, Campbell GP, Perez-Perez GI, Blaser MJ. Purification and characterization of urease from *Helicobacter pylori*. *J Biol Chem* 1990; 265: 9464-9.
24. Austin JW, Doig P, Stewart M, Trust TJ. Macromolecular structure and aggregation states of *Helicobacter pylori* urease. *J Bacteriol* 1991; 173: 5663-7.

25. Labigne A, Cussac V, Courcoux P. Shuttle cloning and nucleotide sequences of *Helicobacter pylori* genes responsible for urease activity. *J Bacteriol* 1991; 173: 1920-31.
26. Mai UE, Perez-Perez GI, Wahl LM, Wahl SM, Blaser MJ, Smith PD. Soluble surface proteins from *Helicobacter pylori* activate monocytes/macrophages by lipopolysaccharide-independent mechanism. *J Clin Invest* 1991; 87: 894-900.
27. Mai UE, Perez-Perez GI, Allen JB, Wahl SM, Blaser MJ, Smith PD. Surface proteins from *Helicobacter pylori* exhibit chemotactic activity for human leukocytes and are present in gastric mucosa. *J Exp Med* 1992; 175: 517-25.
28. Ghiara P, Marchetti M, Blaser MJ, Tummuru MKR, Cover TL, Segal ED, Tompkins LS, Rappuoli R. Role of the *Helicobacter pylori* virulence factors vacuolating cytotoxin, CagA, and urease in a mouse model of disease. *Infect Immun* 1995; 63: 4154-60.
29. Telford JL, Ghiara P. Prospects for the development of a vaccine against *Helicobacter pylori*. *Drugs* 1996; 52: 799-804.
30. Suerbaum S, Josenhans C, Labigne A. Cloning and genetic characterization of the *Helicobacter pylori* and *Helicobacter mustelae* flaB flagellin genes and construction of *H. pylori* flaA- and flaB-negative mutants by electroporation-mediated allelic exchange. *J Bacteriol* 1993; 175: 3278-88.
31. Josenhans C, Labigne A, Suerbaum S. Comparative ultrastructural and functional studies of *Helicobacter pylori* and *Helicobacter mustelae* flagellin mutants: both flagellin subunits, FlaA and FlaB, are necessary for full motility in *Helicobacter* species. *J Bacteriol* 1995; 177: 3010-20.
32. Macchia G, Massone A, Burroni D, Covacci A, Censini S, Rappuoli R. The Hsp60 protein of *Helicobacter pylori*: structure and immune response in patients with gastroduodenal diseases. *Mol Microbiol* 1993; 9: 645-52.
33. Suerbaum S, Thiberge J, Kansau I, Ferrero RL, Labigne A. *Helicobacter pylori* hspA-hspB heat -shock gene cluster: nucleotide sequence, expression, putative function and immunogenicity. *Mol Microbiol* 1994; 14: 959-74.
34. Radcliff RJ, Hazell SL, Kolesnikow T, Doidge C, Lee A. Catalase, a novel antigen for *Helicobacter pylori* vaccination. *Infect Immun* 1997; 65: 4668-74.
35. Ghiara P, Covacci A, Telford JL, Rappuoli R. *Helicobacter pylori*: pathogenic determinants and strategies for vaccine design. In: Kaufmann SHE, ed. *Concepts in Vaccine Development*. Berlin: Walter de Gruyter & Co, 1996: 459-96.
36. Boren T, Falk P, Roth KA, Larson G, Normark S. Attachment of *Helicobacter pylori* to human gastric epithelium mediated by blood group antigens. *Science* 1993; 262: 1892-5.
37. Falk PG, Bry L, Holgersson J, Gordon JI. Expression of a human alpha-1,3/4-fucosyltransferase in the pit cell lineage of FVB/N mouse stomach results in production of Le(b)-containing glycoconjugates: a potential transgenic mouse model for studying *Helicobacter pylori* infection. *Proc Natl Acad Sci USA* 1995; 92: 1515-9.
38. Ilver D, Amqvist A, Ogren J, Frick IM, Kersulyte D, Incecick ET, Covacci A, Engstrand L, Borel T. *Helicobacter pylori* adhesin binding fucosylated histo-group antigens revealed by retagging. *Science* 1998; 279: 373-7.
39. Moren AP, Helander IM, Kosunen TU. Compositional analysis of *Helicobacter pylori* rough-form lipopolysaccharides. *J Bacteriol* 1992; 174: 1370-7.
40. Muotiala A, Helander IM, Pyhala L, Kosunen TU, Moran AP. Low biological activity of *Helicobacter pylori* lipopolysaccharide. *Infect Immun* 1992; 60: 1714-6.
41. Aspinall GO, Monteiro MA, Pang H, Walsh EJ, Moran AP. O antigen un the lipopolysaccharide of *Helicobacter pylori* NCTC 11637. *Carbohydrate Lett* 1994; 1: 151-6.
42. Negrini R, Lisato L, Zanella I, Cavazzini L, Gullini S, Villanacci V, Poiesi C, Albertini A, Ghielmi S. *Helicobacter pylori* infection induces antibodies cross-reacting with human gastric mucosa. *Gastroenterology* 1991; 101: 437-45.

43. Wirth HP, Yang MQ, Karita M, Blaser MJ. Expression of the human cell surface glycoconjugates Lewis X and Lewis Y by *Helicobacter pylori* isolates is related to cagA status. *Infect Immun* 1996; 64: 4598-605.
44. Chen M, Lee A, Hazell S. Immunisation against gastric helicobacter infection in a mouse/ *Helicobacter felis* model [letter]. *Lancet* 1992; 339: 1120-1.
45. Marchetti M, Aricò B, Burroni D, Figura N, Rappuoli R, Ghiara P. Development of a mouse model of *Helicobacter pylori* infection that mimics human disease. *Science* 1995; 267: 1655-8.
46. Marchetti M, Rossi M, Giannelli V, Giuliani MM, Pizza M, Censini S, Covacci A, Massari P, Pagliaccia C, Manetti R, Telford JLT, Douce G, Dougan G, Rappuoli R, Ghiara P. Protection against *Helicobacter pylori* infection in mice by intragastric vaccination with *H. pylori* antigens is achieved using a nontoxic mutant of *E. coli* heat labile enterotoxin (LT) as adjuvant. *Vaccine* 1998; 16: 33-7.
47. Michetti P, Corthesy-Theulaz I, Davin C, Haas R, Vaney AC, Heitz M, Bille J, Kraehenbuhl JP, Saraga E, Blum AL. Immunization of BALB/c mice against *Helicobacter felis* infection with *H. pylori* urease. *Gastroenterology* 1994; 107: 1002-11.
48. Ferrero RL, Thiberge JM, Huerre M, Labigne A. Recombinant antigens prepared from the urease subunits of *Helicobacter* spp: evidence of protection in a mouse model of gastric infection. *Infect Immun* 1994; 62: 4981-9.
49. Ferrero RL, Thiberge M, Kansau I, Wusher N, Huerre M, Labigne A. Immunisation with *H. pylori* heat shock protein A (HspA) and urease subunit B (UreB) affords total protection against *H. felis* infection in mice. *Gut* 1995; 37 (Suppl. 1): A51.
50. Ghiara P, Rossi M, Marchetti M, DiTommaso A, Vindigni C, Ciampolini F, Covacci A, Telford JLT, DeMagistris MT, Pizza M, Rappuoli R, DelGiudice G. Therapeutic intragastric vaccination against *Helicobacter pylori* in mice eradicates an otherwise chronic infection and confers protection against reinfection. *Infect Immun* 1997; 65: 4996-5002.
51. Douce G, Trucotte C, Cropley I, Roberts M, Pizza M, Domenighini M, Rappuoli R, Dougan G. Mutants of *Escherichia coli* heat-labile toxin lacking ADP-ribosyltrasferase activity act as nontoxic, mucosal adjuvants. *Proc Natl Acad Sci USA* 1995; 92: 1644-8.
52. Pizza M, Fontana MR, Giuliani MM, Domenighini M, Magagnoli C, Gianelli V, Nucci D, Hol W, Manetti R, Rappuoli R. A genetically detoxified derivative of heat-labile *Escherichia coli* enterotoxin induces neutralizing antibodies against the A subunit. *J Exp Med* 1994; 80: 2147-53.
53. Doidge C, Gust I, Lee A, Buck F, Hazell S, Manne U. Therapeutic immunisation against *Helicobacter* infection. *Lancet* 1994; 343: 914-5.
54. Corthesy-Theulaz I, Porta N, Glauser M, Saraga E, Vaney AC, Haas R, Kraehenbuhl JP, Blum AL, Michetti P. Oral immunization with *Helicobacter pylori* urease B subunit as a treatment against *Helicobacter* infection in mice. *Gastroenterology* 1995; 109: 115-21.
55. Cuenca R, Blanchard TG, Czinn SJ, Nedrud JG, Monath TP, Lee CK, Redline RW. Therapeutic immunization against *Helicobacter mustelae* in naturally infected ferrets. *Gastroenterology* 1996; 110: 1770-5.
56. Kreiss C, Buclin T, Cosma M, Corthesy-Theulaz I, Michetti P. Safety of oral immunisation with recombinant urease in patients with *Helicobacter pylori* infection. *Lancet* 1996; 347: 1630-1.
57. Lycke N, Tsuji T, Holmgren J. The adjuvant effect of *Vibrio cholerae* and *Escherichia coli* heat-labile enterotoxins is linked to their ADP-ribosyltyransferase activity. *Eur J Immunol* 1992; 22: 2277-81.

Recent advances in the pathogenesis of gastrointestinal bacterial infections.
P. Rampal, P. Boquet, eds. John Libbey Eurotext, Paris © 1998, pp. 25-35.

Progress and problems with vaccination against *Helicobacter pylori*

Irène Corthésy-Theulaz

Department of Internal Medicine, Division of Gastroenterology, Centre Hospitalier Universitaire Vaudois, CH 1011 Lausanne, Switzerland

Why develop a vaccine for *Helicobacter?*

Over half of the world's population is persistently infected with *Helicobacter pylori*. Although all infected individuals have chronic active gastritis, only a minority of these patients develop severe gastrointestinal diseases, including peptic ulcers [1]. The remaining patients exhibit few overt signs of infection but the underlying chronic active gastritis is a significant risk factor for gastric cancer (reviewed in [2]). The organism is susceptible to antimicrobial therapy but antibiotic resistance is emerging (reviewed in [3]) and it is unlikely that antibiotics and altered practices in prevention will be sufficient to eliminate this infection. The development of a safe and effective vaccine, offering the opportunity to treat as well as prevent infection, would thus be a significant achievement to eliminate many severe gastroduodenal diseases [4]. This chapter summarizes the immunobiology of the infection, the vaccines tested so far and the strategies for successful vaccination against *H. pylori*.

Immunobiology of *Helicobacter* infection

Gastric infection by *H. pylori* induces immunoglobulins G (IgG) and A (IgA) immune responses detectable both locally and in the serum of the infected host (reviewed in [5]). The natural immune response to *H. pylori* is characterized by the presence of $CD4^+$ T cells which express mainly a T helper type 1 phenotype (Th1), associated with the production of INF-γ [6-9]. These cells have been shown to participate to the development of the inflammatory response to the infection [9, 10]. It appears then that the natural response, instead of clearing the infection, rather sustains inflammation. Indeed IgG antibodies directed against *H. pylori* have been shown to crossreact with the gastric mucosa [11-13] and systemic immunization of piglets with *H. pylori* antigens resulted in increased inflammation of the gastric mucosa [14]. Similar immune responses were observed in the animal models of *Helicobacter* infection, but as in humans, they were not followed by the disappearance of the infection [15-17].

In theory, the failure of the immune system to clear the infection could be the result of three types of mechanisms. First, the immune effectors may be unable to act on the pathogen (deficient transport of immune effectors across the gastric mucosa, inability of the immune effectors to act in the acidic environment of the stomach or ability of *H. pylori* to escape immune effectors). However, the observation that oral immunization can prevent and, in some instances, cure *H. felis* and *H. pylori* infections rules out this assumption. Second, the immune response may be down-regulated in order to avoid further damage to the host. Third, the immune response may be inadequate (inadequate antigen sampling, stimulation of inappropriate immune effectors). Recently, selective inhibition of Ii-dependent antigen presentation by *H. pylori* toxin VacA has been demonstrated, suggesting that indeed *Helicobacter* is capable of modifying antigen sampling and presentation [18].

Mucosal vaccines against *Helicobacter*

A vaccine approach to prevent or treat *H. pylori* infection was first rejected by the scientific community based on the observation that natural immunity was unable to cure or prevent *Helicobacter* infection and chronic atrophic gastritis. Animal studies, however, have established that immunization with *Helicobacter* whole cell extracts or purified components is able to prevent infection, and more importantly, can clear preexisting infections.

Vaccine candidates

Several vaccines for the prevention or the treatment of *Helicobacter* infection, including whole cell bacterial preparations, purified components, or recombinant proteins have been tested with respect to safety and efficacy in animal models and, for one of them, in clinical trials.

Whole cell vaccines

Whole cell bacterial preparations, inactivated by sonication, were the first vaccines tested [15]. Vaccines based on uncharacterized antigen preparations of *H. pylori*, however, are associated with high costs of production, difficulties of standardization, and a high potential for side effects [9]. This latter point is exemplified by the observation that lipopolysaccharides (LPS) of *H. pylori*, expressing Lewis y, Lewis x and Lewis H type I antigens [11], trigger in mice and humans cross-reactive antibodies that may play a role in gastric damage [19]. This explains why major efforts have been directed towards the identification of *H. pylori* antigens as candidate vaccines.

Subunit antigens

Protective antigens already identified include urease, cytotoxin (VacA), two heat-shock proteins (HspA and HspB), and catalase. The recent availability in the public domain of the entire genome of *H. pylori* should boost the identification of more vaccine antigens.

Urease. Urease is a ~ 550 kDa hexameric molecule composed of two subunits (27 kDa UreA and 62 kDa UreB estimated from the amino-acid sequence). The urease operon consists of nine accessory genes necessary for the proper assembly and function of the enzyme [20]. Immunization of mice with native or recombinant apoenzyme (urease A and B structural subunits), or UreB subunit in conjunction with a mucosal adjuvant prevents [21-23] or cures [24] *Helicobacter* infection. Urease is highly conserved among various *Helicobacter* species [20] and is the best characterized antigen with its value as a protective and curative antigen being confirmed by numerous studies in mice, ferrets, cats, and non-human primates [25-30].

In a double-blind, placebo-controlled phase I clinical trial, oral administration of enzymatically inactive recombinant urease was found to be well tolerated by *H. pylori*-infected asymptomatic adults without changing the course of the infection, as expected, due to the absence of a mucosal adjuvant [31]. More recently, the safety and immunogenicity of recombinant *H. pylori* urease were tested when given with a mucosal adjuvant, the heat-labile enterotoxin of *E. coli* (LT). This latter study confirmed the safety of urease. In addition, urease given with LT induced an immune response and a reduction of the density of gastric *H. pylori* infection, an indication that vaccination may lead to cure of human *H. pylori* infection [32].

VacA. The cytotoxin (VacA) is a ~ 87 kDa molecule that induces vacuolization in several cell lines; it is not expressed in all *H. pylori* isolates, although the gene is present in all *H. pylori* strains (reviewed in [33]). Cytotoxic activity is more prevalent in isolates from patients with peptic ulcers [34]. Orogastric immunization with purified *H. pylori* VacA, together with LT, protects and cures mice against infection by VacA/CagA$^+$ *H. pylori* strains [35, 36]. VacA-based vaccines will not cure or prevent infection with CagA$^-$ strains (40-50% of *H. pylori* strains) which retain their oncogenic potential. However, they could be excellent candidates in any vaccine including other antigens common to all strains.

Chaperones. Chaperones are conserved proteins that contribute to the proper folding of proteins and their assembly into oligomeric structures. They also bind to cellular proteins and protect them against denaturation during stress conditions. Two chaperones, HspA and HspB (heat shock proteins) homologous to GroES and GroEL, respectively, have been identified in *H. pylori* [37]. HspA is involved in the oligomerization of urease. Recombinant *H. pylori* HspA was shown to confer protective immunity in the *H. felis* mouse model [38]. Combining *H. pylori* HspA and UreB with cholera toxin protected mice as efficiently as whole-cell preparations. The use of heat shock proteins, however, as vaccine candidates could induce adverse autoimmune reactions due to the high degree of conservation among the members of the heat shock family and to the expression of *H. pylori*-like chaperones in gastric epithelial cells [12]. Autoimmunity, however, has not been documented in animals immunized with HspA.

Catalase. *H. pylori* catalase is a tetramer with a subunit Mr of 50,000 [39, 40]. It is normally an intracellular oxygen radical scavenging enzyme [41] but might be present on the surface of *H. pylori*. Administration of recombinant catalase together with cholera toxin was shown to protect mice against *H. felis* or *H. pylori* infection [42].

Novel vaccine candidates. Surface proteins, such as adhesins, or exported virulence factors may represent alternatives to the existing vaccines. Cloning strategies to selectively identify surface exposed or secreted proteins have been developed that should facilitate the identification of novel vaccine candidates [43].

Design of an effective vaccine for *Helicobacter*

The difficulty in designing an efficient mucosal vaccine for *Helicobacter* is due to our limited understanding of crucial steps in mucosal immunity, which include the sampling and presentation of antigens in mucosal tissues (reviewed in [44]), and the control of the homing program of memory and effector cells in mucosal lymphoid tissues [45]. These steps are involved in the host response to *Helicobacter* infection and in protective and/or therapeutic immunity induced upon mucosal vaccination.

Vaccine sampling/route of immunization

So far in all preclinical and clinical trials, *Helicobacter*-specific vaccines were administered by the oral route. It is not yet known where the vaccines are sampled. All mucosal surfaces, including those of the airways, the gut and the genital tract, are able to sample antigens and take up vaccines [46] triggering both local and systemic immune responses. There are two major sampling mechanisms *via* dendritic cells or M cells. Dendritic or Langerhans cells in stratified epithelia of the upper digestive and the lower genital tracts take up antigens and transport them to distant (vagina) or local (tonsils) organized lymphoid tissue. Dendritic cells are also present in simple epithelia, for instance in the colon or in the lower respiratory tract [44]. Whether dendritic cells play a major role in uninfected gastric mucosa is yet not known. In mice, the gastric dendritic cells express only a restricted repertoire of dendritic cell markers [47] and it is not clear whether they are present in non infected human gastric mucosa. In simple epithelia, specialized resident epithelial cells, the so-called M cells, in the follicle-associated epithelium (FAE) over mucosal-associated lymphoid tissue (MALT) are able to take up and transport antigens and microorganisms into the underlying lymphoid tissue. The stomach corpus and antrum do not contain FAE and M cells, and hence probably do not sample antigens *via* M cells at least in the absence of *Helicobacter* infection. In *Helicobacter* infected stomachs, however, the bacteria induce MALT [48]. Whether the overlying epithelium contains M cells remains to be established. The induction of MALT, FAE and M cells by microorganisms has been demonstrated in germ free mice, which contain only one or two Peyer's patches [49]. Clearly gastrointestinal epithelial tissues are highly plastic structures which appear to be regulated by a three way interaction between the epithelium, the lymphoid cells, and the microorganisms. It is therefore conceivable that vaccine sampling in *H. pylori*-infected (therapeutic vaccine) or in non-infected stomach (prophylactic vaccine) is different. The identification of the sites where sampling of *H. pylori* antigens and vaccines takes place will help to better design efficient vaccines.

In mice, intranasal or rectal immunizations elicited stronger protection against gastric *Helicobacter* infections than oral immunization ([30] and unpublished results). In humans, the oral and rectal routes of immunization were found to be safe and their importance in eliciting mucosal immune responses in various mucosal compartments already recognized [50, 51] but the optimal route to elicit a response able to protect the gastric mucosa has yet to be determined.

Importance of the adjuvant

In all successful vaccination protocols, mucosal adjuvants, *i.e.* cholera toxin (CT) or *E. coli* labile toxin (LT) had to be added in order to elicit protection or eradication. The use of enterotoxins in humans is restricted because of their side effects (diarrhea). Detoxified adjuvants such as attenuated LT and CT [35, 52, 53] obtained by different genetic interventions on the moiety carrying ADP-ribosyltransferase activity might be promising but their detoxification often alters their immunogenic properties [54] and there is too little data to date on their use in humans to predict their efficacy. There is no clear understanding of the early effects of the toxins on the local (and draining) mucosal lymphoid tissues. This is especially true in the critical areas of antigen presentation, T cell activation, and cytokine production. One of the postulated mechanisms of CT *in vivo* is the inhibition of certain mucosal T cell functions and alteration of the regulatory environment in gut-associated lymphoid tissue [55].

T cell response

Regarding the cellular immune response, several lines of evidence indicate that a Th2 phenotype is associated with protection from infection [10, 56]. Protection or cure indeed correlates with elevated Th2 responses in spleen lymphocytes [56]. In live carrier mediated immunization, we also observed a Th2 response which was characterized by IL-10 secretion rather than IL-4 [57]. Recently, Mohammadi *et al.* isolated splenic lymphocytes from mice immunized with a *H. felis* sonicate plus cholera toxin and challenged with *Helicobacter*. They demonstrated that adoptive transfer of these cells or of antigen specific Th1 or Th2 cell lines exacerbated gastric inflammation in recipients [10]. No effect on bacterial load was observed in recipients of bulk spleen cells from infected mice or recipients of Th1 cell lines. In contrast, recipients showed a reduction in bacterial load when either a Th2 cell line or bulk cells from immunized/challenged mice were adoptively transferred.

The fact that splenic immune cells or a Th2 cell line isolated from immunized mice were able, upon transfer into naive mice, to enable the recipient animals to maintain a lower level of infection is certainly encouraging but the exacerbation of the gastric inflammation is worrying and certainly not desirable for an efficient vaccine. These experiments underline once more the need to use a defined antigen or a combination of defined antigens rather than a whole bacterial sonicate containing multiple uncharacterized antigens with potentially deleterious effects.

Effectors in the gastric mucosa

Since *H. pylori* is a non-invasive pathogen, the immune effectors must gain access to the gastric mucosal surface in order to exert their function. The identity of the immune effectors implicated in the protective or therapeutic activity of the vaccines has not yet been elucidated. Specific secretory IgAs have long been thought to be the appropriate effectors against infection by *Helicobacter*. The protective potential of sIgA is supported by a study in Gambia, in which babies breast-fed by *H. pylori* infected mothers were protected against infection during the entire lactation period [58]. On the other hand, *H. pylori*-specific secretory IgA antibodies are found in secretions of infected individuals, but they are inefficient to clear an established infection. Nedrud and co-workers immunized IgA deficient mice and demonstrated that IgAs were not absolutely necessary as effectors [59]. However, these mice had higher titers of gastric IgM which could have compensated for the lack of IgA considering that IgM can be secreted by the same mechanisms as IgA. These experiments do not rule out a role of secretory IgAs in protection, but suggest that other effectors can be just as effective in the absence of secretory IgAs. A correlation between the presence of *Helicobacter*-specific IgA antibodies and protection was reported in outbred mice immunized with urease apoenzyme [22] but not with urease B subunit [23]. No correlation was found either between sIgA titers and protection in mice immunized with Hsp proteins [38]. In another report, protective properties were attributed to local specific IgGs instead of IgAs [60].

Secretory IgAs might thus not be the sole effectors and it is likely that an array of complementary effectors is necessary to be effective against *Helicobacter*. The involvement of other immune cells such as macrophages and granulocytes deserves attention.

Safety issues

Adverse reactions have been observed in inbred or outbred mice immunized with *H. felis* sonicates or *H. pylori* urease with inflammatory infiltrate appearing in immunized mice after challenge [9, 22, 23, 61].

Epithelial changes consisting of parietal cell loss and hyperplasia of the epithelium were observed [23, 28]. Antimicrobial triple therapy significantly decreased the degree of gastritis and epithelial alteration in the stomach, indicating that residual bacteria might be responsible for the persistent lymphocytic infiltration [28]. Mohamadi *et al.* analyzed the infiltrate over time and postulated a delayed-type hypersensitivity-like reaction elicited by bacterial challenge [9]. A growing body of evidence suggests that a Th1 response promotes changes in the intergrity and the function of the epithelium, thereby enhancing the deleterious effects of luminal acid and pepsin; such a response may be responsible for the postimmunization gastritis [10].

Alternate vaccination strategies

The lack of a mucosal adjuvant which can be safely used in humans has led to the investigation of alternate vaccination strategies that would not require the use mucosal adjuvants. Our group has been interested in two new vaccination strategies; DNA vaccination and antigen delivery by live carriers.

DNA vaccination, consisting of intramuscular injections of naked DNA encoding for a specific antigen leads to specific humoral and cellular responses against the antigen. The exact mechanism that generates a specific response is unknown. Both T helper 1 and 2 responses have been observed after DNA vaccination with several antigens. The factors influencing the response towards each type of response are still being investigated. DNA vaccination of mice with *H. pylori* urease B genes caused a significantly lower degree of infection when compared to the non-immunized group, irrespective of the antibody response [62].

Antigen delivery by attenuated live vaccine carrier represents another alternative to mucosal adjuvants. Mucosal immunization of mice with recombinant attenuated *Salmonella* expressing the two structural subunits of *H. pylori* urease protects mice from *Helicobacter* [57, 63].

What remains to be done to obtain an efficacious anti-*H. pylori* vaccine?

In summary, mucosal immunization resulting in stimulation of the mucosa-associated immune system appears in all animal studies as a prerequisite for protection/cure.

The limited human evidence supports this concept but suggests that the level of stimulation of the immune system obtained in humans with urease plus LT was too low to lead to a clearance of the infection. There is now an urgent need to define reliable immunological markers of protection in order to improve vaccination strategies. Once those are defined, it will be then possible to select the appropriate mucosal adjuvants without gastrointestinal toxicity and the optimal routes of administration, and to design vaccines combining several protective epitopes in order to ensure broader efficacy without side effects.

References

1. Blaser MJ. *Helicobacter pylori* and the pathogenesis of gastroduodenal inflammation. *J Infect Dis* 1990; 161: 626-33.
2. Wisniewski RM, Peura DA. *Helicobacter pylori*: beyond peptic ulcer disease. *Gastroenterologist* 1997; 5: 295-305.
3. Megraud F, Occhialini A, Doermann HP. Resistance of *Helicobacter pylori* to macrolides and nitroimidazole compounds. The current situation. *J Physiol Pharmacol* 1997; 48: 25-38.
4. Michetti P. Vaccine against *Helicobacter pylori*: fact or fiction? *Gut* 1997; 41: 728-30.
5. Genta RM. The immunobiology of *Helicobacter pylori* gastritis. *Semin Gastrointest Dis* 1997; 8: 2-11.
6. Fan XJ, Chua A, Shahi CN, Mc Devitt J, Keeling PWN, Kelleher D. Gastric T lymphocyte responses to *Helicobacter pylori* in patients with *H. pylori* colonisation. *Gut* 1994; 35: 1379-84.
7. Karttunen R, Andersson G, Poikonen K, Kosunen TU, Karttunen T, Juutinen K, Niemela S. *Helicobacter pylori* induces lymphocyte activation in peripheral blood cultures. *Clin Exp Immunol* 1990; 82: 485-8.
8. Karttunen R, Karttunen T, Ekre HPT, MacDonald TT. Interferon gamma and interleukin 4 secreting cells in the gastric antrum in *Helicobacter pylori* positive and negative gastritis. *Gut* 1995; 36: 341-5.
9. Mohammadi M, Czinn S, Redline R, Nedrud J. *Helicobacter*-specific cell-mediated immune responses display a predominant Th1 phenotype and promote a delayed-type hypersensitivity response in the stomachs of mice. *J Immunol* 1996; 156: 4729-38.
10. Mohammadi M, Nedrud J, Redline R, Licke N, Czinn S. Murine CD4 T-cell response to *Helicobacter* infection: TH1 cells enhance gastritis and TH2 cells reduce bacterial load. *Gastroenteroloy* 1997; 133: 1846-57.
11. Appelmelk BJ, Simoons-Smit I, Negrini R, Moran AP, Aspinall GO, Forte JG, De Vries T, Quan H, Verboom T, Maaskant JJ, Ghiara P, Kuipers EJ, Bloemena E, Tadema TM, Townsend RR, Tyagarajan K, Crothers Jr. JM, Monteiro MA, Savio A, De Graaff J. Potential role of molecular mimicry between *Helicobacter pylori* lipopolysaccharide and host Lewis blood group antigens in autoimmunity. *Infect Immun* 1996; 64: 2031-40.
12. Engstrand L, Scheynius A, Pahlson C. An increased number of gamma/delta T-cells and gastric epithelial cell expression of the groEL stress-protein homologue in *Helicobacter pylori*-associated chronic gastritis of the antrum. *Am J Gastroenterol* 1991; 86: 976-80.
13. Negrini R, Lisato L, Zanella I, Cavazzini L, Gullini S, Villanacci V, Poiesi C, Albertini A, Ghielmi S. *Helicobacter pylori* infection induces antibodies cross-reacting with human gastric mucosa. *Gastroenterology* 1991; 101: 437-45.
14. Eaton KA, Krakowka S. Chronic active gastritis due to *Helicobacter pylori* in immunized gnotobiotic piglets. *Gastroenterology* 1992; 103: 1580-6.

15. Chen M, Lee A, Hazell S. Immunisation against gastric helicobacter infection in a mouse/ *Helicobacter felis* model. *Lancet* 1992; 339: 1120-1.
16. Fox JG, Blanco M, Murphy JC, Taylor NS, Lee A, Kabok Z, Pappo J. Local and systemic immune responses in murine *Helicobacter felis* active chronic gastritis. *Infect Immun* 1993; 61: 2309-15.
17. Fox JG, Correa P, Taylor NS, Lee A, Otto G, Murphy JC, Rose R. Helicobacter mustelae-associated gastritis in ferrets. An animal model of *Helicobacter pylori* gastritis in humans. *Gastroenterology* 1990; 99: 352-61.
18. Molinari M, Salio M, Galli C, Norais N, Rappuoli R, Lanzavecchia A, Montecucco C. Selective inhibition of Ii-dependent antigen presentation by *Helicobacter pylori* toxin VacA. *J Exp Med* 1998; 187: 135-40.
19. Claeys D, Faller G, Appelmek BJ, Negrini R, TK. The gastric H,K-ATPase is a major autoantigen in chronic *Helicobacter pylori* gastritis with body mucosa atrophy. *Gastroenterology* 1998 (in revision).
20. Mobley HLT, Island MD, Hausinger RP. Molecular biology of microbial ureases. *Microbiol Rev* 1995; 59: 451-80.
21. Ferrero RL, Thiberge JM, Huerre M, Labigne A. Recombinant antigens prepared from the urease subunits of *Helicobacter* spp: evidence of protection in a mouse model of gastric infection. *Infect Immun* 1994; 62: 4981-9.
22. Lee CK, Weltzin R, Thomas Jr. WD, Kleanthous H, Ermak TH, Soman G, Hill JE, Ackerman SK, Monath TP. Oral immunization with recombinant *Helicobacter pylori* urease induces secretory IgA antibodies and protects mice from challenge with *Helicobacter felis*. *J Infect Dis* 1995; 172: 161-72.
23. Michetti P, Corthesy-Theulaz I, Davin C, Haas R, Vaney AC, Heitz M, Bille J, Kraehenbuhl JP, Saraga E, Blum AL. Immunization of BALB/c mice against *Helicobacter felis* infection with *Helicobacter pylori* urease. *Gastroenterology* 1994; 107: 1002-11.
24. Corthesy-Theulaz I, Porta N, Glauser M, Saraga E, Vaney AC, Haas R, Kraehenbuhl JP, Blum AL, Michetti P. Oral immunization with *Helicobacter pylori* urease B subunit as a treatment against *Helicobacter* infection in mice. *Gastroenteroloy* 1995; 109: 115-21.
25. Batchelder M, Fox JG, Monath T, Yan L, Attardo L, Georakopoulos K, Li X, Marini R, Shen Z, Pappo J, Lee C. Oral vaccination with recombinant urease reduces gastric *Helicobacter pylori* colonization in the cat. *Gastroenterology* 1996; 110: A58.
26. Cuenca R, Blanchard TG, Czinn SJ, Nedrud JG, Monath TP, Lee CK, Redline RW. Therapeutic immunization against *Helicobacter mustelae* in naturally infected ferrets. *Gastroenterology* 1996; 110: 1770-5.
27. Dubois A, Lee C, Fiala N, Kleanthous H, Monath T. Immunization against natural *Helicobacter pylori* infection in Rhesus monkeys. *Gut* 1996; 39: A43-A40.
28. Ermak TH, Ding R, Ekstein B, Hill J, Myers GA, Lee CK, Pappo J, Kleanthous HK, Monath TP. Gastritis in urease-immunized mice after *Helicobacter felis* challenge may be due to residual bacteria. *Gastroenterology* 1997; 113: 1118-28.
29. Marchetti M, Arico B, Burroni D, Figura N, Rappuoli R, Ghiara P. Development of a mouse model of *Helicobacter pylori* infection that mimics human disease. *Science* 1995; 267: 1655-8.
30. Weltzin R, Kleanthous H, Guirakhoo F, Monath TP, Lee CK. Novel intranasal immunization techniques for antibody induction and protection of mice against gastric *Helicobacter felis* infection. *Vaccine* 1997; 15: 370-6.
31. Kreiss C, Buclin T, Cosma M, Corthesy-Theulaz I, Michetti P. Safety of oral immunisation with recombinant urease in patients with *Helicobacter pylori* infection. *Lancet* 1996; 347: 1630-1.

32. Michetti P, Kreiss C, Kotloff K, Porta N, Blanco JL, Corthésy-Theulaz I, Losonsky G, Nichols R, Stolte M, Monath T, Ackerman S, Blum AL. Oral immunization with recombinant urease and LT adjuvant in *Helicobacter pylori*-infected humans. *Gastroenterology* 1997; 112: A1042.
33. Cover TL, Berg DE, Blaser MJ. VacA and the *cag* pathogenicity island of *H. pylori*. In: Ernst PB, Michetti P, Smith PD, eds. *The Immunobiology of* H. pylori. *From Pathogenesis to Prevention*. Philadelphia: Lippincott-Raven, 1997: 75-90.
34. Telford JL, Ghiara P, Dell Orco M, Commanducci M, Burroni D, Bugnoli M, Tecce MF, Censini S, Covacci A, Xiang Z, Papini E, Montecucco C, Parente L, Rappuoli R. Gene structure of the *Helicobacter pylori* cytotoxin and evidence of its key role in gastric disease. *J Exp Med* 1994; 179: 1653-8.
35. Ghiara P, Rossi M, Marchetti M, Di Tommaso A, Vindigni C, Ciampolini F, Covacci A, Telford J, De Magistris M, Pizza M, Rappuoli R, Del Giudice G. Therapeutic intragastric vaccination against *Helicobacter pylori* in mice eradicates an otherwise chronic infection and confers protection against reinfection. *Infect Immun* 1997; 65: 4996-5002.
36. Manetti R, Massari P, Marchetti M, Magagnoli C, Nuti S, Lupetti P, Ghiara P, Rappuoli R, Telford JL. Detoxification of the *Helicobacter pylori* cytotoxin. *Infect Immun* 1997; 65: 4615-9.
37. Dunn BE, Roop RMI, Sung CC, Sharma SA, Perez-Perez GI, Blaser MJ. Identification of a cpn60 Heat Shock Protein homolog from *Helicobacter pylori*. *Infect Immun* 1992; 60: 1946-51.
38. Ferrero RL, Thiberge JM, Kansau I, Wuscher N, Huerre M, Labigne A. The GroES homolog of *Helicobacter pylori* confers protective immunity against mucosal infection in mice. *Proc Natl Acad Sci USA* 1995; 92: 6499-503.
39. Hazell SL, Evans Jr. DJ, Graham DY. *Helicobacter pylori* catalase. *J Gen Microbiol* 1991; 137: 57-61.
40. Odenbreit S, Wieland B, Haas R. Cloning and genetic characterization of *Helicobacter pylori* catalase and construction of a catalase-deficient mutant strain. *J Bacteriol* 1996; 178: 6960-7.
41. Mori M, Suzuki H, Suzuki M, Kai A, Miura S, Ishii H. Catalase and superoxide dismutase secreted from *Helicobacter pylori*. *Helicobacter* 1997; 2: 100-5.
42. Radcliff FJ, Hazell SL, Kolesnikow T, Doidge C, Lee A. Catalase, a novel antigen for *Helicobacter pylori* vaccination. *Infect Immun* 1997; 65: 4668-74.
43. Odenbreit S, Till M, Haas R. Optimized BlaM-transposon shuttle mutagenesis of *Helicobacter pylori* allows the identification of novel genetic loci involved in bacterial virulence. *Mol Microbiol* 1996; 20: 361-73.
44. Kraehenbuhl JP, Hopkins SA, Kerneis S, Pringault E. Antigen sampling by epithelial tissues: implication for vaccine design. Behring Inst. Mitt., 1997: 24-32.
45. Farstad IN, Halstensen TS, Kvale D, Fausa O, Brandtzaeg P. Topographic distribution of homing receptor on B and T cells in human gut-associated lymphoid tissue: relation of L-selectin and integrin alpha 4 beta 7 to naive and memory phenotypes. *Am J Pathol* 1997: 150: 187-99.
46. Neutra MR, Pringault E, Kraehenbuhl JP. Antigen sampling across epithelial barriers and induction of mucosal immune responses. *Annu Rev Immunol* 1996; 14: 275-300.
47. Soesatyo M, Biewenga J, Kraal G, Sminia T. The localization of macrophage subsets and dendritic cells in the gastrointestinal tract of the mouse with special reference to the presence of high endothelial venules. An immuno- and enzyme- histochemical study. *Cell Tissue Res* 1990; 259: 587-93.
48. Stolte M, Eidt S. Lymphoid follicles in antral mucosa: immune response to *Campylobacter pylori*. *J Clin Pathol* 1989; 42: 1269-71.
49. Savidge TC, Smith MW, James PS, Aldred P. *Salmonella*-induced M-cell formation in germ-free mouse Peyer's patch tissue. *Am J Pathol* 1991; 139: 177-84.

50. Kozlowski PA, Cu-Uvin S, Neutra MR, Flanigan TP. Comparison of the oral, rectal, and vaginal immunization routes for induction of antibodies in rectal and genital tract secretions of women. *Infect Immun* 1997; 65: 1387-94.
51. Nardelli-Haefliger D, Kraehenbuhl JP, Curtiss RR, Schodel F, Potts A, Kelly S, De Grandi P. Oral and rectal immunization of adult female volunteers with a recombinant attenuated *Salmonella typhi* vaccine strain. *Infect Immun* 1996; 64: 5219-24.
52. Douce G, Fontana M, Pizza M, Rappuoli R, Dougan G. Intranasal immunogenicity and adjuvanticity of site-directed mutant derivatives of cholera toxin. *Infect Immun* 1997; 65: 2821-8.
53. Pizza M, Fontana MR, Giuliani MM, Domenighini M, Magagnoli C, Giannelli V, Nucci D, Hol W, Manetti R, Rappuoli R. A genetically detoxified derivative of heat-labile *Escherichia coli* enterotoxin induces neutralizing antibodies against the A subunit. *J Exp Med* 1994; 180: 2147-53.
54. Guidry JJ, Cardenas L, Cheng E, Clements JD. Role of receptors binding in toxicity, immunogenicity, and adjuvanticity of *Escherichia coli* heat-labile enterotoxin. *Infect Immun* 1997; 65: 4943-50.
55. Elson CO, Holland SP, Dertzbaugh MT, Cuff CF, Anderson AO. Morphologic and functional alterations of mucosal T cells by cholera toxin and its B subunit. *J Immunol* 1995; 154: 1032-40.
56. Saldinger PF, Porta N, Launois P, Louis JA, Waanders GA, Michetti P, Blum AL, Corthesy-Theulaz I. Mucosal immunization of BALB/c mice with *Helicobacter* urease B induces a T helper 2 response not seen during infection with *Helicobacter*. Submitted.
57. Corthesy-Theulaz I, Hopkins S, Bachmann D, Saldinger PF, Porta N, Haas R, Yan ZX, Meyer T, Bouzourène H, Blum AL, Kraehenbuhl JP. Mice are protected from *Helicobacter pylori* infection by nasal immunization with attenuated *Salmonella typhimurium phoPc* expressing urease A and B subunits. *Infect Immun* 1998; 66: 581-6.
58. Thomas JE, Austin S, Dale A, McClean P, Harding M, Coward WA, Weaver LT. Protection by human milk IgA against *Helicobacter pylori* infection in infancy. *Lancet* 1993; 342: 121.
59. Nedrud J, Blanchard T, Czinn S, Harriman GR. Orally-immunized IgA deficient mice are protected against *H. felis* infection. *Gut* 1996 (Suppl. 2), A45.
60. Ferrero RL, Thiberge JM, Labigne A. Local immunoglobulin G antibodies in the stomach may contribute to immunity against *Helicobacter* infection in mice. *Gastroenterology* 1997; 113: 185-94.
61. Pappo J, Thomas Jr. WD, Kabok Z, Taylor NS, Murphy JC, Fox JG. Effect of oral immunization with recombinant urease on murine *Helicobacter felis* gastritis. *Infect Immun* 1995; 63: 1246-52.
62. Corthesy-Theulaz I, Corthesy B, Bachmann D, Porta N, Vaney AC, Saraga E, Michetti P, Kraehenbuhl JP, Blum AL. Naked DNA immunization against *Helicobacter* infection. *Gastroenterology* 1996; 110.
63. Gomez-Duarte OG, Lucas B, Yan ZX, Panthel K, Haas R, Meyer TF. Protection of mice against gastric colonization by *Helicobacter pylori* by single oral dose immunization with attenuated *Salmonella typhimurium* producing urease subunits A and B. *Vaccine* 1998; 16: 460-71.

Immune system
in the gastrointestinal tract

Recent advances in the pathogenesis of gastrointestinal bacterial infections.
P. Rampal, P. Boquet, eds. John Libbey Eurotext, Paris © 1998, pp. 39-55.

Organization and regulation of intestinal immunity

Jiry Mestecky

Departments of Microbiology and Medicine, University of Alabama at Birmingham, Birmingham, AL, USA

Mucosal surfaces represent the major interface between the host and the environment. Thus, it is not surprising that most pathogens invade through or infect mucosal surfaces [1]. The host has clearly evolved a number of defense mechanisms to deal with microbes in general and pathogens in particular. One of the most important of these is the mucosal immune system. This compartment of the immune system, quantitatively the largest, is marked by a number of distinguishing features that are unique to its specialized role.

The antigenic challenge to the intestinal immune system is enormous. It has been estimated that the number of microbial cells in the body, most of them in the intestine, exceeds the total number of cells in the body [2]. One can add to these bacterial antigens the abundant antigens present in food and drink. Exactly how the intestinal mucosal system deals with this challenge is not yet known; however, it is apparent that the mucosal immune system is in a constant state of response, as witnessed by the large number of plasma cells present throughout the intestine and by studies on germ-free animals in whom the mucosal lymphoid tissue is poorly developed [3].

Intestinal lymphoid compartments

Lymphoid cells in the intestine are found in three histologically and functionally distinct compartments, usually in the lymphoepithelial structures – Peyer's patches (PP), lamina propria, and in the intraepithelial localization.

Lymphoepithelial inductive sites

PP are organized lymphoid aggregates with one or more lymphoid follicles that extend from the epithelial layer into the lamina propria, and sometimes the submucosa. Although PP are visible, macroscopic structures, clustered in certain regions such as the ileum in man, analogous small lymphoid follicles are dispersed abundantly throughout the intestine in humans and some other species [4]. PP and these small follicles together comprise gut-associated lymphoid tissue (GALT). PP differ from other peripheral lymphoid tissues by the lack of afferent lymphatics, but do have efferent lymphatics. Instead of afferent lymphatics, they have a specialized epithelium that actively pinocytoses material present in the intestinal lumen and delivers it *via* trancytosis and exocytosis into the follicle *(figure 1)*. Distinguishing features of this specialized follicle-associated epithelium or FAE include a relative lack of goblet cells and the presence of M or microfold cells that lack polymeric immunoglobulin receptor (pIgR) (see below) and alkaline phosphatase [5]. The M cell serves as an important first step in the induction of intestinal immune responses, but relatively little is known about the factors determining its generation or function. Soluble proteins, viruses, bacteria, protozoa, and innert particles (*e.g.*, loposomes, and microspheres) have all been taken up by M cells. Some organisms such as *Salmonella* exploit this feature, using M cells as a portal of entry into the body. M cell uptake of *Salmonella* and particles such as microspheres is being exploited to deliver vaccine antigens into GALT. Human M cells have the potential to take up the antigen and delivery it directly to the lymphocytes infiltrating the dome epithelium; no evidence of antigen presentation by M cells exists.

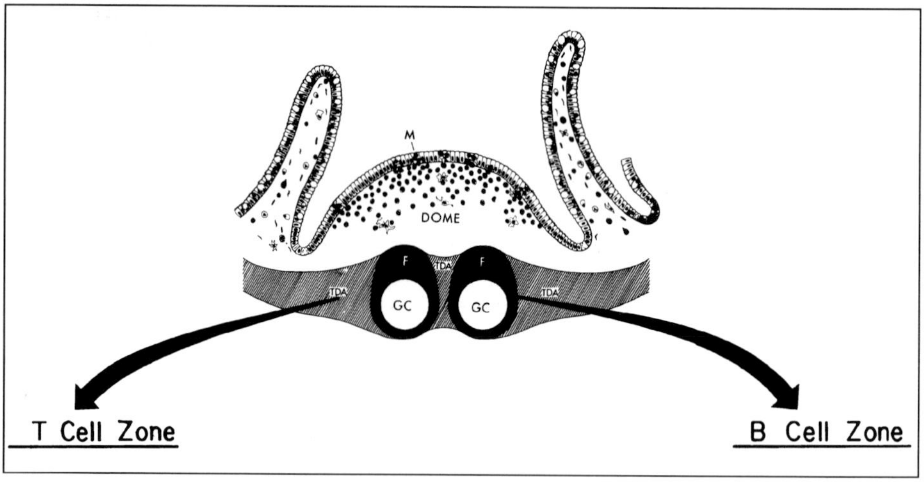

Figure 1. General morphology of Peyer's patches: M: microfold cell in the dome region involved in phagocytosis and pinocytosis of lumenal antigens; F: lymphoid follicle; GC: germinal center; TDA: thymus-dependent area.

Consistent with this active antigen uptake by the specialized dome epithelium, PP and related lymphoid follicles serve as sites for the induction of mucosal immune responses. It is now recognized that the PP contains all the cells needed for immune induction, *i.e.*, B cells, T cells, and antigen-processing and -presenting cells (macrophages, dendritic cells, and follicular dendritic cells). These cell types are structured in B-cell-dependent and T-cell-dependent areas similar to other peripheral lymphoid tissues. B cells predominate in the lymphoid follicles, whereas T cells predominate in the interfollicular areas and beneath the dome epithelium; macrophages appear to be scattered both beneath the dome epithelium and in the follicles [4]. Quantitatively, B cells predominate in the PP of adult animals constituting some 60 to 70% of total cells, while T cells, including both $CD4^+$ and $CD8^+$ cells, comprise about 20% of the total. An important feature of PP cells is that they consist of precursor rather than effector cells. For example, although the PP contains many B cells, few plasma cells are present, even after extensive immunization. The same appears to be true for cytotoxic T cells (CTL). One explanation is that differentiating B cells and T cells leave PP and migrate to the gut and other lymphoid tissues (see below). A second important feature of PP is that the induction of immune responses there is highly dependent on the route of antigen exposure. PP respond predominantly, if not exclusively, to antigen present in the intestinal lumen, that is, antigen transported by M cells.

GALT and analogous structures present in the respiratory tract in some species (bronchus-associated lymphoid tissue, BALT) are sites in which there is preferential induction of IgA responses, an important function considering that IgA is the major immunoglobulin at mucosal surfaces. PP cells are enriched for B cell precursors of IgA-producing plasma cells relative to other lymphoid tissues [6], particularly for IgA B cell precursors recognizing antigens present in the intestine. The mechanism for this preferential expression of IgA by PP B cells is not clear, but microenvironmental-B-cell interactions, the effects of an unusual switch T cell, the effects of a specialized dendritic cell, or the expression of cytokines such as tumor growth factor-β (TGF-β) in PP are possible explanations. T cells regulate B-cell differentiation by secreting a variety of cytokines *(figure 2)*; such T cells are present in the PP as well [7].

The discovery that antigen-stimulated GALT or BALT are the source of antigen-sensitized and IgA-committed plasma cell precursors that populate remote mucosal tissues and glands has led to the concept of a common mucosal immune system (CMIS) [8], in which an antigen exposure at one mucosal surface contributes cells to help protect remote mucosal sites as well *(figure 3)*. For example, immunization of the gut through GALT can generate a mucosal response in tears, milk, saliva, and genital tract secretions. This had led to a renewed interest in the development of oral vaccines to protect non-intestinal mucosal sites. Priming for a mucosal response *via* the intestine is convenient and effective, but an optimal immunity at distant mucosal sites may also require local exposure of that mucosal surface to the antigen. In fact, the CMIS may comprise certain subcompartments so that optimal vaginal immune responses occur after rectal immunization, whereas optimal upper respiratory immune responses occur after nasopharyngeal or BALT immunization.

In regard to the intestine, lymphoid cells constitute approximately 25% of the cells; therefore the intestine is a major lymphoid organ [9]. As mentioned above, the mucosal immune system of the gut is organized into several interconnecting compartments representing either inductive or effector sites. Inductive sites consist of PP and isolated lymphoid follicles; effector sites consist of the lamina propria and IEL. The mesenteric lymph nodes, although outside the intestine proper, are frequently considered a fourth compartment. These different cell compartments are distinguished not only by differences in physical location and structure, but also by the types and functions of cells present within them.

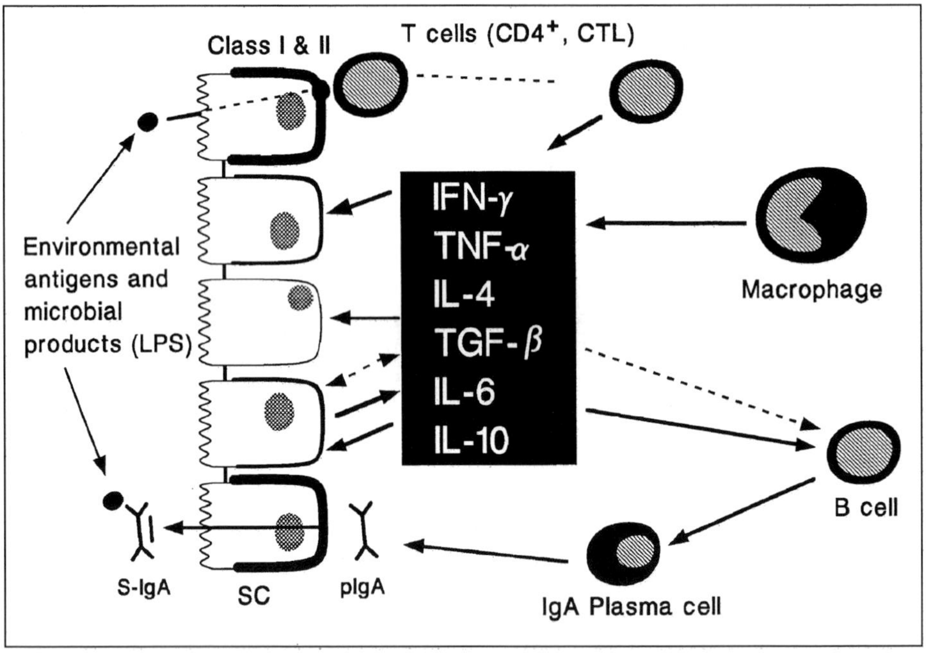

Figure 2. Participation of epithelial, lymphoid, and myeloid cells in cytokine networks of mucosal tissues. Epithelial cells are in constant contact with antigen and bioactive products of microbes, which activate epithelial cells to produce a variety of cytokines that can interact with mucosal immune cells. Epithelial cells also can express class II MHC molecules and thus potentially act as antigen-presenting cells to induce either immunity or tolerance. In turn, mucosal immune cells produce local cytokines that act on epithelial cells. The physiological consequences for epithelial cell function are still being defined, but these cytokines can increase expression of certain molecules such as MHC class II molecules and pIgR (SC), as well as to further enhance epithelial cell cytokine production.

Lamina propria lymphocytes

The intestinal lamina propria contains an abundance of B cells, plasma cells, T cells, and macrophages as well as a lesser number of other cell types such as eosinophils, mast cells and dendritic cells [9]. The intestinal lamina propria is the only site in the body where large numbers of plasma cells are present continuously. Approximately 70% to 90% of the plasma cells in the intestine produce IgA. In humans, the next most common isotype produced is IgM, representing 5% to 15%, followed by IgG, representing only 3% to 5%. IgE and IgD plasma cells are infrequent.

Plasma cells are terminally differentiated, end stage cells whose half-life is approximately 5-10 days, indicating that there must be a dynamic, continuous repopulation of lamina propria B cells. The proliferation and differentiation of B cells appears to be regulated by cytokines produced by a broad spectrum of resident cell types, particularly T cells, but including also macrophages and epithelial cells [7] *(figure 2)*. With respect to differentiation of mucosal B cells into IgA plasma cells, interleukin-5 (IL-5), IL-6, IL-10 and TGF-β play prominent roles. Recent studies suggest that these cytokines are derived not only from T cells, but also from epithelial cells which can produce IL-6, IL-10 and TGF-β [7-12].

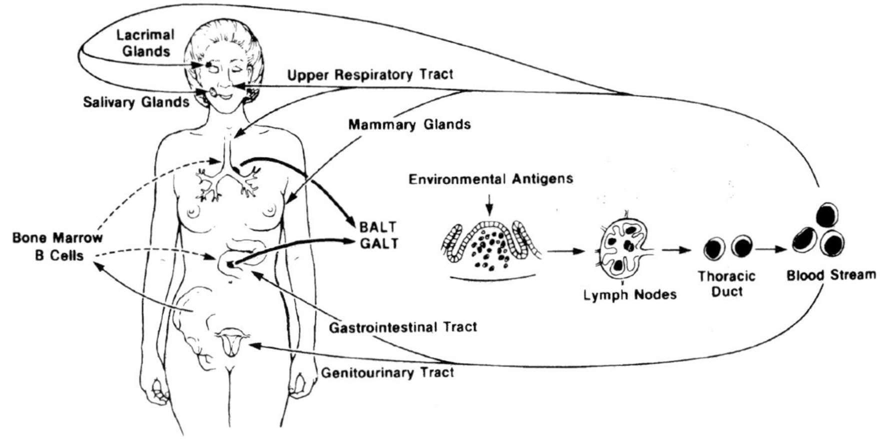

Figure 3. Diagram of the common mucosal immune system in humans. Lymphoid cells, presumably from the bone marrow, enter the inductive sites (*e.g.*, PP) through post-capillary high endothelial venules. Under the local influence of T cells, epithelial cells, and accessory cells (dendritic cells) they express surface IgA. Environmental antigens enter PP through pinocytotic and phagocytic M cells and interact with resident accessory, T, and B cells. IgA-committed and antigen-sensitized B cells and lymphoblasts leave PP and enter the regional lymph nodes, then the lymph and circulation. Finally, such cells populate various exocrine glands and mucosa-associated tissues, where terminal differentiation into IgA-secreting plasma cells occurs. BALT apparently plays a role analogous to that of GALT. It is thought that tonsils may also contribute to the pool of precursor cells that populate the upper respiratory and digestive tract.

It is possible to isolate human lamina propria lymphocytes and study their functions *in vitro*. In such isolates, cells of B lymphocyte lineage comprise some 15% to 40% of the total cells with IgA-producing cells predominating. Considerable numbers of T cells are present also, ranging from 40% to 90%. Macrophages make up about 10% of lamina propria isolates, and eosinophils and mast cells from 1% to 3%. Interestingly, cells with neither B cell or T cell markers, that is, null cells, and cells with natural killer (NK) cell markers seem to be deficient in the intestinal lamina propria, although cells capable of lymphokine-activated killer (LAK) activity are well represented.

The ability to isolate lamina propria cells from human and primate intestine has allowed lamina propria T cells to be characterized. Approximately two-thirds of lamina propria T cells are $CD4^+$ and one-third are $CD8^+$, which is similar to their ratio in peripheral blood. However, lamina propria T cells differ in substantial ways from peripheral blood T cells. Most of the lamina propria T cells have the $CD45RO^+$ $CD45RA^-$ phenotype characteristic of memory cells, whereas the converse is true for peripheral blood T cells. Lamina propria T cells are in a higher state of activation based on expression of IL-2Rα chain, HLA-DR molecules, transferrin receptors, and CD98 (an activation molecule recognized by the monoclonal antibody 4F2). Upon activation lamina propria T cells produce greater amounts of cytokines such as IL-2, IL-4, IL-5 and interferon-g (IFN-γ), which is consistent with their increased helper activity for B cell responses [13]. Human lamina propria T cells have diminished proliferative responses to stimulation *via* the CD3/TCR complex but respond normally to stimulation *via* CD2 or CD28. There appears to be a soluble mediator produced in the intestinal mucosa that down regulates the CD3/TCR pathway of T cell activation. T cells with markers consistent with cytolytic T-cell function are present in the lamina propria, and functional cytolytic activity has been demonstrated in intestinal lymphocytes by redirected lysis assays. Whether such cytolytic activity is brought into play during normal intestinal immune responses is unclear, but such cells could be important in host defense against certain pathogens.

Intraepithelial lymphocytes (IEL)

Lymphocytes that are physically located within the epithelial layer, or IELs, comprise one out of every 6-10 cells in the epithelium [14]. The cellular composition of this compartment is different from that in either the PP or the lamina propria. Plasma cells are not present, and B cells are absent or infrequent. The predominant cell type in small intestinal IEL is the $CD8^+$ T cell, and in most mouse strains, about half bear $\gamma\delta$ T-cell receptors and the other half $\alpha\beta$ T-cell receptors. In mice IEL are quite heterogenous based on expression of CD8 isoforms, Thy1, CD5, and on cell density. Whether similar heterogeneity exists in human IEL is unclear. Analysis of human IEL TCR gene expression shows evidence of oligocloanality; similar analysis of murine IEL TCR expression has not been done. In contrast to mice or chickens, T$\gamma\delta$ cells are a minor component in human IELs, most of which are TCR$\alpha\beta^+$, $CD8^+$, $CD45RO^+$. Most existing data on IEL come from studies done on small intestinal isolates. It is interesting therefore that mouse colon IEL have been found to consist mainly of $CD4^+$, TCR$\alpha\beta^+$ T cells, revealing previously unsuspected regional differences within the intestinal immune system. Whether similar regional differences exist for the lamina propria compartment is unknown. The environment in the small bowel and colon is dramatically different and so it should not be surprising that the mucosal immune system of these two sites is also different. It is quite possible that these regional differences in mucosal lymphoid populations is an important aspect of host defense against the enteric flora and against pathogens but no direct evidence of this exists at present.

IEL T$\alpha\beta$ cells appear to originate in the PP and traffic to the epithelium *via* the lamina propria but there is evidence as well for a thymic-independent lineage of T cells in small intestinal IELs. The origin of these cells, which bear the CD8$\alpha\alpha$

isoform and are $CD5^-$, remains unclear. In many species, a large proportion of the IELs contain granules that stain metachromatically and resemble mast cell granules, but contain little or no histamine.

The function of IELs in host defense remains unclear. First, IELs have full cytotoxic capabilities including NK, ADCC, and T cell cytotoxicity. Because IEL increase in number after roundworm infestations, they might serve a cytotoxic function directed primarily at parasites. Second, IELs are increased in experimental graft *versus* host disease, prompting the suggestion that an increase in IELs may be a marker for cell-mediated immune responses in the intestine. Third, IELs might defend the epithelium against viral infections by local secretion of IFN-γ, and perhaps by direct cytotoxicity. They may produce other cytokines that may influence enterocyte functions. Although we know little about their precise function *in vivo*; IELs are situated in a site that would render them exposed to a variety of antigenic stimuli and thus they likely play an important role in mucosal host defense.

Mucosal lymphocyte trafficking

Lymphocytes induced in the GALT exit *via* efferent lymphatics and enter into mesenteric lymph nodes where they may undergo further division and differentiation [10]. From there they travel *via* the thoracic duct into the circulation and are dispersed widely in the body [11]. However, these cells selectively accumulate back (or "home") to the intestine and other mucosal sites such as the lactating breast, salivary and lacrimal gland and perhaps genitourinary tissues, *i.e.*, tissue of CMIS *(figure 3)*. The migration of IgA-producing cells from GALT to the lactating breast is an important mechanism that provides specific secretory IgA antibodies in mother's milk to protect the suckling newborn against the microbes with which it is most likely to be colonized. This dissemination of antigen-sensitized and IgA-committed cells from inductive sites to remote effector sites has important implications for the design of vaccines that would provide protective immunity at mucosal surfaces, the most frequent portals of entry of infectious agents. In order to populate the lamina propria of the intestine or remote secretory glands, such cells must exit the circulation. Numerous studies suggest that specific interactions between receptors on lymphocytes and those on the endothelial cells of specialized high endothelial venules (HEV) regulate the selective distribution of lymphocytes to secondary lymphoid tissues [10]. The molecular mechanisms of cell trafficking is an area of active research. A number of molecules important in cell migration into mucosae have been identified to date. These lymphocyte molecules and their respective endothelial cell ligands include LFA-1 (CD18/CD11a) binding to ICAM-1/ICAM-2, VLA-4 binding to VCAM-1, and CD44 binding to a 58- to 66-kDa molecule. Recent biochemical characterization of one mucosal vascular addressin that is selectively expressed on HEV of mucosal lymphoid organs and on lamina propria venules reveals that this receptor displays features comon to members of the immunoglobulin supergene family. This receptor, designated the mucosal addressin cell adhesion molecule (MAdCAM1) is composed of three immunoglobulin domains and a 37-amino-acid region localized between the second and third domains. This region is rich in serine and threonine, which are potential glycosylation sites for O-linked carbohydrates. Interestingly, the first and the second domains display sequences homologous to the human VCAM-1 molecule and the third domain to the CH2 domain of human IgA1; the intervening serine/threonine-rich region exhibits structural features characteristic of mucins. This unusual carbohydrate may play a role in lymphocyte binding and migration.

The entry of cells into a tissue such as the intestine is a critical component of mucosal immunity as well as of mucosal inflammation. In regard to the latter, inflammatory cytokines increase the expression of endothelial cell ICAM-1 and ELAM-1 during intestinal inflammation, thus facilitating entry of larger numbers of cells into inflammatory sites. The entry of non-specific inflammatory cells into the intestine *via* these molecules is an important element of host defense against infectious pathogens, particularly early during infection before specific immunity has been triggered.

Mucosal immunoglobulins and their contribution to defense mechanisms

Approximately 8 g of immunoglobulins (Igs) are produced per day in a 75 kg human. When individual isotypes are considered, roughly 60% of all Ig produced is of the IgA isotype (70 mg/kg/day), 30% of IgG (35 mg/kg/day) 7% of IgM (8 mg/kg/day), and small amounts of IgD and IgE [16]. However, human sera contain relatively low levels of IgA as compared to IgG, because more than half of the IgA produced is selectively transported by a receptor-mediated mechanism into external secretions [16]. Furthermore, the half-life of human serum IgA is considerably shorter due to its fast catabolism (5-6 days for IgA and 20-24 days for IgG) *(figure 4).*

Structure of secretory IgA

In contrast to almost all animal species that produce IgA, human IgA molecules are more heterogenous: there are two subclasses (IgA1 and IgA2) as well as two characteristically distributed molecular forms – monomeric (m) and polymeric (p) IgA. In serum, mIgA1 predominates over mIgA2 while in external secretions almost exclusively polymeric forms of approximately equal proportions of IgA1 and IgA2 are found *(figure 4).* The different molecular forms of human IgA display different biological activities including interactions with IgA receptors and antigens [18].

Human IgA occurs in multiple genetic forms encoded on chromosome 14. IgA1 and IgA2 have been identified by serologic and structural studies [7, 18], also in hominoid primates (*e.g.* chimpanzee and gorilla); in other species (except Lagomorphs), only one IgA isotype is present.

Primary amino acid and carbohydrate structures of human IgA of both subclasses have been determined [7, 18]. There are surprisingly few differences in the amino acid sequences in the constant region of $\alpha 1$ and $\alpha 2$ chains, except for the hinge region, which in the $\alpha 1$ chain is highly susceptible to unique IgA1-specific proteases produced by several bacterial species that frequently colonize mucosal surfaces and

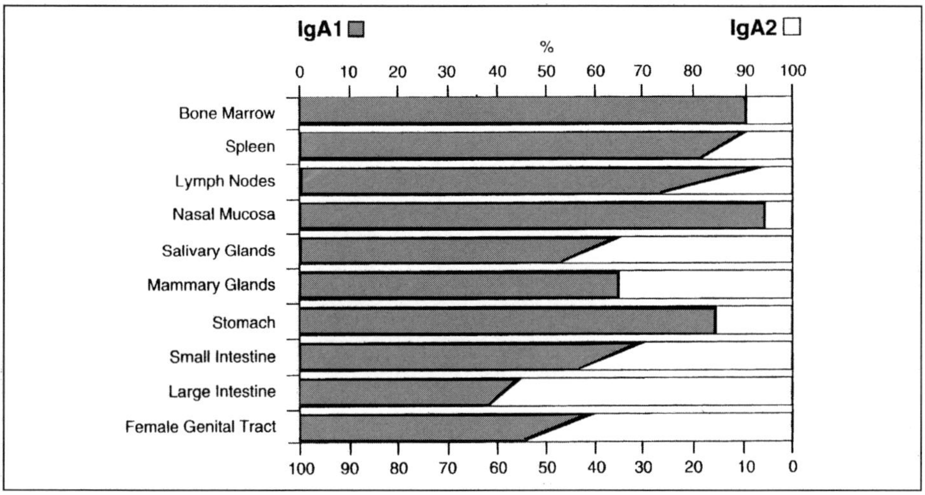

Figure 4. Estimated contributions of systemic (bone marrow, lymph nodes, and spleen) and mucosa-associated compartments of the IgA system to mucosal secretions and the circulatory pools. A large amount of predominantly mIgA produced in bone marrow is catabolized in the liver and other sites; in humans IgA from the circulation contributes little to the pool of IgA found on mucosal surfaces. Most IgA produced at secretory sites is selectively transported by a pIgR-dependent pathway into external secretions; approximately 10% enters the circulatory pool.

can cause localized or systemic diseases [19]. Interestingly, the gene segment encoding the hinge region represents a recent insertion into the α chain gene.

The cells that produce IgA1 or IgA2 also display a characteristic tissue distribution [20]. In the bone marrow, approx. 90% of the cells are IgA1-positive and thus mirror the intravascular distribution of this subclass; on the other hand, mucosal tissues and glands contain variable proportions of IgA1 and IgA2 cells, depending on the anatomic origin of the tissue. Although IgA1 cells predominate in most of these mucosal tissues, the relative contribution of IgA2 cells is more pronounced; in the large intestine and the female genital tract, the IgA2 cells outnumber the IgA1 cells *(figure 5)*. Although the reason for the typical tissue distribution of IgA1 and IgA2 cells is not known, it is possible that environmental antigens present in a given locale may be responsible for the IgA subclass-specific expansion of cells (see below).

In pIgA, an additional small glycoprotein, J chain, is present; it is attached to the penultimate cysteine residues of two α chains. With respect to pIgA and mIgA, the former molecular form is principally produced by plasma cells distributed in the mucosal tissues and glands where almost all of the IgA-positive cells express J chain. In contrast, IgA-positive plasma cells in normal human bone marrow secrete almost exclusively mIgA.

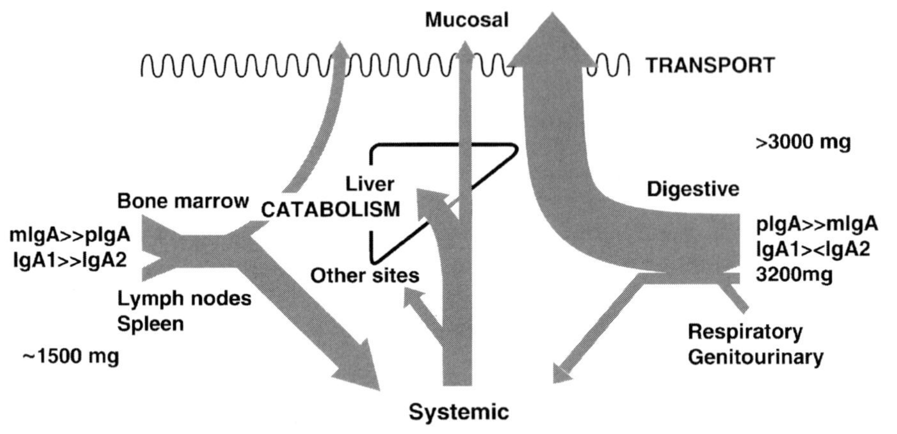

Figure 5. Distribution (in %) of IgA1- and IgA2-producing cells in systemic and mucosal tissues in humans.

Receptors involved in the distribution of IgA molecules and their functional significance

IgA interacts with surface membrane receptors on a broad spectrum of morphologically and functionally different cell types. As a consequence of these interactions, a variety of biologically important phenomena occur, including the selective transport of pIgA through epithelial cells and hepatocytes into external secretions and bile, removal of IgA-containing immune complexes (IgA-IC) by hepatocytes and Kupffer cells, hepatic catabolism of IgA, enhanced phagocytosis of IgA-coated bacteria by mucosal polymorphonuclear leukocytes and macrophages, and degranulation of eosinophils ([16] also see below). The receptors involved in IgA binding by various cells have been only partially characterized with respect to their properties, distribution, and relative biological importance. The best characterized receptor, pIgR, is expressed on human and animal epithelial cells covering mucosal surfaces, and on ductal and acinar cells of external secretory glands [21]. pIgR displays Ig domain-like structure and is involved in the binding and extremely efficient transport of J chain-containing pIgA and pIgM.

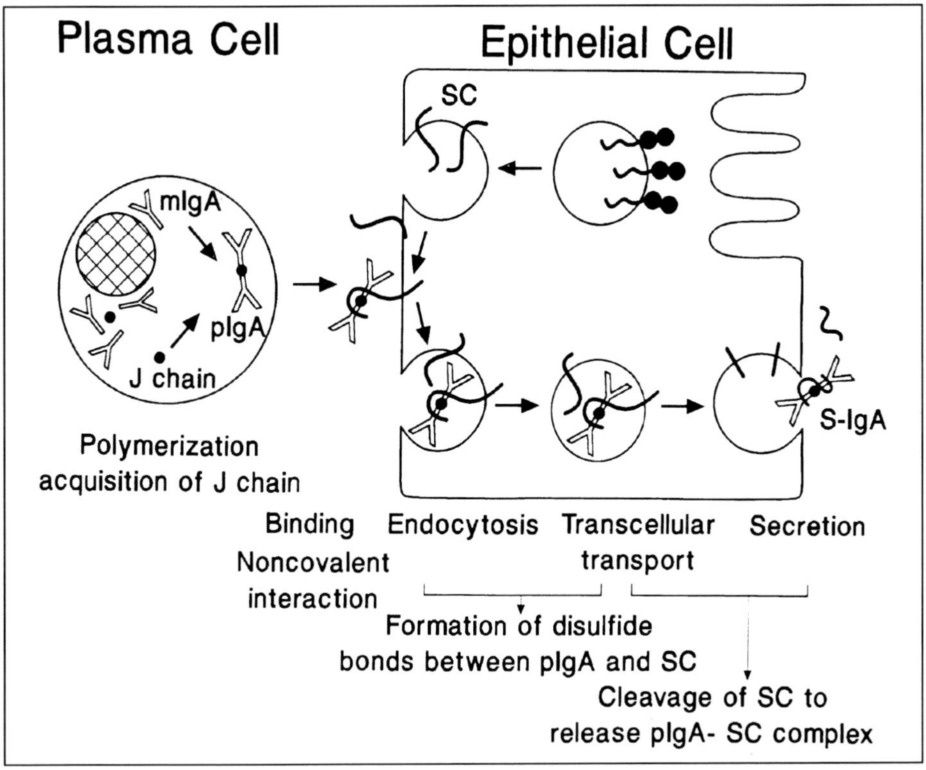

Figure 6. General model of the pIgR(SC)-mediated transport of pIgA through epithelial cells. pIgR produced in the rough endoplasmic reticulum is terminally glycosylated in the Golgi apparatus and transported in vesicles to the basolateral surface of epithelial cells. The cytoplasmic tail of pIgR provides a signal for this targeting. The extracellular SC interacts with the SC-binding site on pIgA. SC-pIgA complexes are internalized in vesicles and subsequently transcytosed with the participation of microtubules to the apical surface of epithelial cells where they fuse with the membrane. Proteolytic cleavage of SC occurs in this location, and S-IgA molecule is released.

Secretory IgA and its transport system

The appearance of large amount of IgA in external secretions, and particularly in the intestinal tract, is the result of complex molecular and cellular interactions that have been studied in great detail [16, 21]. Most plasma cells at mucosal sites produce pIgA in its dimeric and tetrameric forms. Intracellular polymerization of monomers and the incorporation of an additional small glycoprotein J chain within the plasma cell results in the secretion of IgA molecules that can interact with pIgR specific for polymeric immunoglobulins of the IgA and IgM isotypes. This receptor, also called secretory component (SC), which is expressed on the surface of epithelial cells and, in some species on hepatocytes, plays a key role in the selective epithelial transport of IgA. After synthesis in the rough endoplasmic reticulum and heavily glycosylation in the Golgi complex, pIgR reaches and is inserted into the basolateral membrane of the enterocyte, where it acts as a receptor. After the initial interactions of pIgA with pIgR on epithelial cells through noncovalent binding, its first domain binds to the Cα3 domain, and the fifth domain binds covalently to the Cα2 domain. J chain is essential for polymeric IgA to interact with pIgR, probably by inducing conformational changes in IgA that permit SC binding. Following these molecular events, the membrane pIgR-pIgA complex is internalized and transported in vesicles toward the apical surface of the epithelial cells. Once there, these vesicles fuse with the apical membrane. Proteolytic cleavage of pIgR releases the assembled molecule of secretory IgA (S-IgA) into external secretions. pIgR-mediated transport of pIgA represents a unique system of interaction between a receptor and its ligand: pIgR is produced by epithelial cells regardless of the presence of its ligand and is not recycled. Instead, it remains permanently attached to pIgA and confers an increased resistance of S-IgAto proteolytic enzymes in the intestinal tract. The magnitude of selective IgA transport is enormous, comprising 3-5g S-IgA produced and transported each day into the human intestine.

The synthesis and expression of both J chain and SC is regulated by cytokines and hormones [16, 21]: IL-5, IL-2 and possibly IL-6 up regulate J chain synthesis while IL-4, IFN-γ, TNF-α and TGF-β significantly enhance pIgR expression. Thus, the synthesis of all component chains of S-IgA is regulated by cytokines that are locally produced in the intestinal microenvironment.

Functional uniqueness of IgA

Biological functions of S-IgA are summarized in *table I* and described in detail in [22]. Generally, S-IgA alone can neutralize biologically active antigens (*e.g.*, viruses and toxin), interfere with the absorption of protein antigens from the gut lumen, and inhibit the adherence of microorganisms to epithelial cells.

Table I. Effector functions of serum and secretory IgA

Direct
- Neutralization of biologically active antigens (viruses, enzymes, toxins)
- Inhibition of antigen absorption from mucosal membranes (immune exclusion)
- Inhibition of microbial adherence to epithelial cells and tooth surfaces

Indirect
- Enhancement of antibacterial humoral factors in external secretions (lactoferrin and peroxidase system)
- Promotion of phagocytosis by mucosal polymorphonuclear leukocytes and macrophages
- Enhancement of monocyte and lymphocyte-dependent bactericidal activity
- Degraulation of eosinophils
- Anti-inflammatory activity by blockage of IgM-, IgG-, or IgE-mediated reactions and complement activation (chemotaxis, phagocytosis, immune lysis, anaphylaxis and Arthus reactions)
- Clearance of circulating immune complexes by hepatobiliary transport (in some species)
- Antibody-dependent cellular cytotoxicity
- Regulation of T cell activity (induction of IgA-binding factors and possibly interleukins resulting in increased or decreased production of IgA by stimulated B cells)

In contrast to the function of other isotypes of Ig that can be easily demonstrated by dramatic biological reactions (antibody-dependent killing and lysis of prokaryotic and eukaryotic cells, promotion of phagocytosis, anaphylaxis, etc.), the consequences of the union of IgA antibodies with corresponding antigens are more subtle. Generally, this is due to the restricted ability of IgA to use ancillary effector mechanisms such as activation of complement, phagocytosis, and binding to other effector cells.

In contrast with IgM and IgG, IgA antibodies are essentially non-inflammatory in their mode of action, a property that is probably of great importance for the maintenance of the integrity of mucosal surfaces as well as internal tissues.

IgA and complement. The concept that IgA represents a "safe" form of anti-inflammatory antibody is exemplified by the findings that intact native human IgA antibodies fail to activate complement by either major pathway when complexed with antigen, and further that they powerfully interfere with complement activation by IgM and IgG antibodies [23]. The frequently cited ability of IgA to promote turnover of the alternative complement pathway (ACP) on close examination turns out to be due to artificial aggregation or conformational alteration of IgA induced by exposure to denaturing agents during purification, heat, deposition on hydrophobic surfaces, chemical cross-linking or modification, or aberrant synthesis.

IgA and phagocytes. Phagocytes (including monocytes/macrophages, neutrophils and eosinophils) express FcαR, which, at least under certain circumstances is capable of mediating phagocytosis and transducing signals for oxidative metabolism and granule release [23]. FcαR is a heterogeneous receptor that appears to be extensively and variably glycosylated depending in part on the cell type on which it is expressed, and its intracellular connections with signal-transducing systems are beginning to be elucidated. Although FcαR is constitutively expressed on monocytes, neutrophils and eosinophils, it is up-regulated by certain cytokines. Exposure of neutrophils to tumor necrosis factor α (TNF-α) or interleukin (IL)-8 increases surface expression of FcαR and enhances their ability to respond to IgA-opsonized particles [23]. Tissue macrophages appear to express FcαR variably, and it is not known what regulates this expression, nor its functional significance. In the case of neutrophils, which in their resting state appear to respond weakly if at all to IgA-complexed antigen, it can be speculated that enhanced expression of FcαR on exposure to inflammatory or chemotactic cytokines has functional significance within mucosal tissues such as the gut. IL-8 and TNF-α released by epithelial cells exposed to aggressive bacteria attract and activate neutrophils to a site of potential pathogenic challenge, and functional up-regulation of their FcαRs enables them to be effective phagocytes in the IgA-rich environment of the submucosa. It is particularly noteworthy that IgA, and especially S-IgA, when coupled to agarose, is the most potent stimulus for eosinophil degranulation [23]. As eosinophils occur frequently in mucosal tissues and are implicated in defense against metazoan parasites, this may be an important effector activity of IgA. However, further work is necessary in this area, especially using IgA (and S-IgA) antibodies complexed with antigens to model more closely the physiological situation.

Regulation of the intestinal mucosal immune system

Immunity to antigens after intestinal exposure is well documented following natural infections in man and oral immunization regimens in experimental animals. The large quantity of IgA produced in the intestine reflects a continuous and active mucosal immune response to antigens in the environment. The mechanisms by which this response is regulated are currently being defined [24]. Mention has already been made of the helper function of the lamina propria $CD4^+$ T cell. Murine $CD4^+$ T cells in mice can be further subdivided into two types, based on the cytokines that they secrete and thus the functions that they serve *(figure 7)*. Type 1 (Th1) $CD4^+$ cells produce IL-2 and IFN-γ and mediate delayed hypersensitivity responses; type 2 (Th2) $CD4^+$ T cells produce IL-4, IL-5, IL-6 and IL-10 and serve as helper cells for B cell responses [25]. Th1 and Th2 cells reciprocally regulate one another *via* the cytokines IL-10 and IFN-γ *(figure 7)*. The balance between these two subsets may be very important in maintaining mucosal homeostasis and host defense, because the Th1 *vs* Th2 pattern of response in inbred mouse strains can mean death or survival of the host to various infectious agents. The factors which determine whether Th1 or Th2 cells will predominate in the response to a given pathogen are obviously important but as yet not understood. The current notion is that the initial encounter of the microbe with cells of the innate immune system (macrophages, granulocytes, mast cells, etc.) stimulates the production of certain cytokines, namely IL-12 or IL-4, which induce differentiation down the Th1 or Th2 pathway, respectively *(figure 7)*.

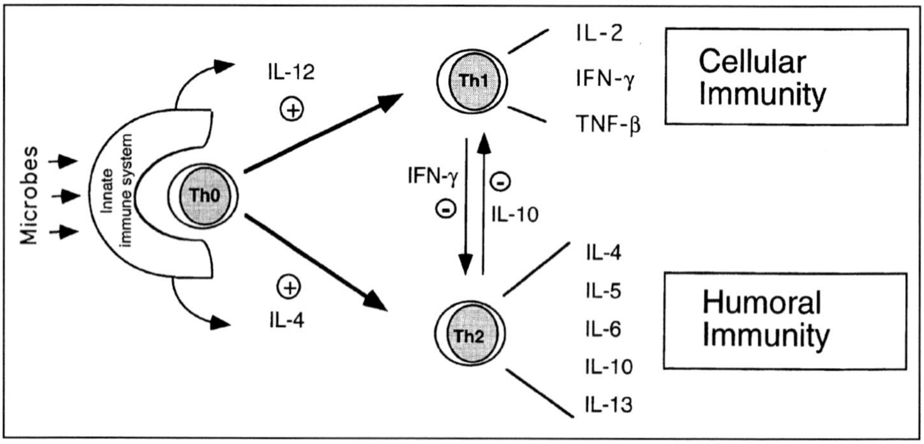

Figure 7. T-cell differentiation pathways induced by microbes. The initial encounter of microbes is with cells of the innate immune system (antigen-presenting cells, mast cells, granulocytes, stromal cells). This system provides a rapid but non specific response. Specific responses are generated by the presentation of microbial antigens by cells of the innate immune system to naive $CD4^+$ T cells (Th0). Depending on the cytokine milieu in the microenvironment, $CD4^+$ Th0 cells differentiate along either or both of two pathways, *i.e.*, into Th1 cells that mediate cellular immune responses or into Th2 cells that mediate humoral immunity. Th1 and Th2 cells are distinguished by their production of certain cytokines as shown. They also produce many other cytokines in common. These two subsets regulate one another through interferon-γ (Th1) and IL-10 (Th2), which inhibit the reciprocal subset. For a given microbe, the predominant pathway stimulated can determine whether the infection results in disease or recovery.

The exact role of Th1 and Th2 cells in the regulation of mucosal immunity is not yet known, however mucosal sites seem to have a propensity for Th2-type responses to antigens. For example, the same antigen (tetanus toxoid) when given parenterally induces predominantly Th1 responses in the spleen, but given orally induces predominantly Th2 responses in the lamina propria. The balance between Th1 and Th2 cells is likely to be an important factor in mucosal host defense toward microbial flora as well as microbial pathogens. The importance of this regulatory balance is illustrated by the development of chronic colitis in mice in whom IL-10 or IL-2, cytokines important in maintaining such T cell subset balance, have been genetically deleted. Much less is known about Th1 and Th2 cells in humans but evidence is emerging that similar T cell subsets are being found in humans with chronic parasitic and mycobacterial diseases.

The feeding of an antigen prior to parenteral immunization can induce a state of systemic unresponsiveness or "oral tolerance" [24, 26] instead of immunity. The factors determining whether immunity or tolerance result from an antigen encounter in the gut are not well understood, but presumably the answer lies in complex regulatory cell interactions within GALT. Oral tolerance has been demonstrated in animals after the feeding of a variety of antigens including proteins, contact allergens, heterologous erythrocytes, and viral hemagglutinin. Some evidence exists that bacterial LPSs may sensitize the mucosal immune system in a manner that predisposes to development of oral tolerance, and to non-specific suppression. Multiple mechanisms of tolerance have been demonstrated, but the most common one is the generation of suppressor $CD8^+$ T cells in GALT. These $CD8^+$ T cells may secrete TGF-β, an inhibitory cytokine, as a mechanism for their suppression. There seems to be differential cellular susceptibility to oral tolerance induction, with Th1 cells being most sensitive, followed by Th2 cells and then B cells. Feeding autoantigens has been used to abrogate or treat experimental autoimmune diseases, and recently trials have begun along a similar line in humans. A recent study has shown that the feeding of a protein antigen to human volunteers did result in T cell, but not B cell, tolerance establishing for the first time that oral tolerance exists in humans [27]. It is unclear whether protein antigens of bacterial origin can induce oral tolerance. Bacterial lipopolysaccharide given together with a non-bacterial antigen increased the degree of oral tolerance to the latter, so the presence of highly stimulatory adjuvant molecules in microbes does not necessarily shift the mucosal response away from a tolerizing one. There have been a dearth of studies in which bacterial antigens have been tested for their ability to induce oral tolerance. The feeding of large amounts of *E. coli* alkaline phosphatase to mice did not result in oral tolerance, but whether this result can be extrapolated is unclear. The factors which determine whether tolerance or immunity occurs after a mucosal encounter with microbial antigens need to be defined. This is clearly an important consideration both for the outcome of any encounter with an intestinal pathogen, as well as for the possible development of oral vaccines against such infectious agents.

References

1. McGhee JR, Mestecky J. In defense of mucosal surfaces. Development of novel vaccines for IgA responses protective at portals of entry for microbial pathogens. *Infect Dis Clin North Am* 1990; 4: 315-41.
2. Savage DC. Microbial ecology of the gastrointestinal tract. *Annu Rev Microbiol* 1977; 31: 107-33.
3. Abrams GD, Bauer H, Sprinz H. Influence of the normal flora on mucosal morphology and cellular renewal in the ileum. *Lab Invest* 1963; 12: 355-64.
4. Bockman DE, Boydston WR, Beezhold DH. The role of epithelial cells in gut-associated immune reactivity. *Ann N Y Acad Sci* 1983; 409: 129-43.
5. Owen RL, Jones AL. Epithelial cell specialization within human Peyer's patches: and ultrastructural study of intestinal lymphoid follicles. *Gastroenterology* 1974; 66: 189-03.
6. Craig SW, Cebra JJ. Peyer's patches: an enriched source of precursors for IgA-producing immunocytes in the rabbit. *J Exp Med* 1971; 134: 188-200.
7. McGhee JR, Mestecky J, Elson CO, Kiyono H. Regulation of IgA synthesis and immune response by T cells and interleukins. *J Clin Immunol* 1989; 9: 175-99.
8. Scicchitano R, Stanisz A, Ernst P, Bienenstock J. A common mucosal immune system revisited. In: Husband AJ, ed. *Migration and homing of lymphoid cells*. Boca Raton: CRC Press, 1988: 1-35, vol 2.
9. Brandtzaeg P. Research in gastrointestinal immunology. State of the art. *Scand J Gastroent* 1985; 20: 137-56.
10. Picker LJ, Butcher EC. Physiological and molecular mechanisms of lymphocyte homing. *Annu Rev Immunol* 1992; 10: 561-91.
11. Phillips-Quaggliata JM, Lamm ME. Lymphocyte homing to mucosal effector sites. In: Ogra PL, Mestecky J, Lamm ME, Strober W, McGhee JR, Bienenstock J, ed. *Handbook of mucosal immunology*. San Diego: Academic Press, 1994: 225-34.
12. Beagley KW, Elson CO. Cells and cytokines in mucosal immunity and inflammation. *Gastroenterol Clin North Am* 1992; 21: 347-66.
13. James SP. Mucosal T-cell function. *Gastroenterol Clin N Am* 1992; 20: 597-12.
14. Ernst PB, Befus AD, Bienenstock J. Leukocytes in the intestinal epithelium: an unusual immunological compartment. *Immunol Today* 1985; 6: 50-5.
15. LeFrancois L. Intraepithelial lymphocytes: Ontogeny. In: Ogra PL, Mestecky J, Lamm ME, Strober W, McGhee JR and Bienenstock J, eds. *Mucosal immunology*, 2nd ed. San Diego, CA: Academic Press, 1998: in press.
16. Mestecky J, Lue C, Russell MW. Selective transport of IgA: cellular and molecular aspects. *Gastroenterol Clin North Am* 1991; 20: 441-71.
17. Underdown BJ, Mestecky J. Mucosal immunoglobulins. In: Ogra PL, Mestecky J, Lamm ME, Strober W, McGhee JR, Bienenstock J, eds. *Handbook of mucosal immunology*. San Diego, CA: Academic Press, 1994: 79-97.
18. Mestecky J, Russell M.W. IgA subclasses. *Monogr Allergy* 1986; 19: 277-301.
19. Kilian M, Reinholdt J, Lomholt H, Poulsen K, Frandsen EVG. Biological significance of IgA1 proteases in bacterial colonization and pathogenesis: critical evaluation of experimental evidence. *Acta Pathol Microbiol Immunol Scand* 1996; 104: 321-38.
20. Kutteh WH, Mestecky J. Concept of mucosal immunology. In: Bronson RA, Alexander NJ, Anderson DJ, Branch DW, Kutteh WH, eds. *Reproductive Immunology*. Cambridge, MA: Blackwell Science, 1996: 28-51.

21. Brandtzaeg P, Krajci P, Lamm ME, Kaetzel CS. Epithelial and hepatobiliary transport of polymeric immunoglobulins. In: Ogra PL, Mestecky J, Lamm ME, Strober W, McGhee JR, Bienenstock J, eds. *Handbook of mucosal immunology*. San Diego, CA: Academic Press, 1994: 113-23.
22. Russell MW, Sibley DA, Nikolova EB, Tomana M, Mestecky J. IgA antibody as a non-inflammatory regulator of immunity. *Biochem Soc Trans* 1997; 25: 466-70.
23. Kilian M, Russell MW. Function of mucosal immunoglobulins. In: Ogra PL, Mestecky J, Lamm ME, Strober W, McGhee JR, Bienenstock J, eds. *Handbook of mucosal immunology*. San Diego, CA: Academic Press, 1994: 127-37.
24. Elson CO. Induction and control of the gastrointestinal immune system. *Scand J Gastroenterol* 1985; 114: 1-15.
25. Mosmann TR, Coffman RL. Th1 and Th2 cells: different patterns of lymphokine secretion lead to different functional properties. *Annu Rev Immunol* 1989; 7: 145-74.
26. Weiner HL. Oral tolerance: immune mechanisms and treatment of autoimmune diseases. *Immunol Today* 1997; 18: 335-43.
27. Husby S, Mestecky J, Moldoveanu Z, Holland S, Elson CO. Oral tolerance in humans. T cell but not B cell tolerance after antigen feeding. *J Immunol* 1994; 152: 4663-70.

Recent advances in the pathogenesis of gastrointestinal bacterial infections.
P. Rampal, P. Boquet, eds. John Libbey Eurotext, Paris © 1998, pp. 57-63.

Follicle-associated epithelium: structure, role in antigen sampling and ontogeny

Jean-Pierre Kraehenbuhl, Lucy Hathaway, Nathalie Debard

Swiss Institute for Experimental Cancer Research and Institute of Biochemistry, University of Lausanne, CH-1066 Epalinges, Switzerland

Organization of mucosal epithelial barriers

The mucosal surfaces of the digestive tract, the airways and the genital tract are covered by epithelia which constitute an efficient physical barrier that allows exchanges between the environment and the internal milieu while at the same time protecting the host from environmental pathogens. The upper digestive tract (oral cavity, pharynx and esophagus) consists of a stratified epithelium while the stomach, and the small and large intestine are covered by a simple epithelium. Similarly, a simple epithelium covers the upper genital tract (uterus and tubes in females and epididyme, vas deferens in males) and a malpighian stratified epithelium is associated with the lower surfaces (vagina and urethra). A pseudostratified epithelium covers the upper airways and a simple epithelium is found in lower respiratory tract.

Stratified epithelia are composed of multiple layers of cells lacking tight junctions but which provide a permeability barrier to ions, small molecules, and macromolecules by secreting a glycoprotein that seals the spaces between the cells and excludes the entry of most infectious microorganisms.

In contrast to stratified epithelia, the intercellular spaces of simple epithelia are sealed by tight junctions that constitute an efficient diffusion barrier. In addition, mucus and luminal cell surface structures, including the glycocalyx, prevent microorganisms contacting and adhering to the plasma membrane. Uptake of macromolecules, particulate antigens, and microorganisms across intact simple epithelia is restricted to the epithelium in close contact with mucosal associated tissue, the follicle-associated epithelium (FAE) which contains specialized cells, the so-called M cells (for review see [1, 2]).

Renewal and differentiation of mucosal epithelia

The mucosal surfaces are continuously exposed to environmental or locally produced hazardous substances (irritants, toxics, toxins, carcinogens). Epithelial cells damaged by these substances are normally rapidly eliminated due to their continuous cell renewal. In mice, for instance, the epithelial cells complete their terminal differentiation within 48-72 hours. This rapid turn-over, which is tightly regulated, prevents the accumulation of DNA lesions which may lead to malignant transformation.

The microflora, which consists of non-pathogenic microorganisms that form complex colonies which survive in the luminal compartment, especially of the digestive tract, despite continuous changes of the environment, can influence the host epithelial cell differentiation programs. They may do so either directly [3] or indirectly by triggering the expression and release of epithelial signaling molecules that recruit migratory host cells, including neutrophils, lymphocytes and monocytes [4, 5]. Disruption of this signaling pathway results in chronic inflammatory responses resembling human inflammatory bowel diseases [6, 7].

The mucosal surfaces are protected against pathogens both by innate and adaptive defense mechanisms [8]. Surveillance of epithelial cell integrity and growth is mediated by specialized lymphocytes which are found within the epithelium, the so-called intraepithelial lymphocytes (IEL) [9]. In the gut, the type of T cell receptor ($\gamma\delta$ or $\alpha\beta$)) and CD8 molecules expressed by IELs varies along the gastrointestinal tract and along the crypt villus axis [10]. IELs have been proposed to play various roles in the gut: elimination of stressed or damaged gastric and intestinal cells, induction of local immune unresponsiveness to food antigens [11], and control of epithelial cell proliferation [12]. There is evidence that IELs recognize non classical MHC class I molecules expressed on intestinal epithelial surfaces [13] suggesting that they play a critical functional role in the regulation of the immune responses to local antigens [14]. They could down-regulate immune cells hence preventing the development of delayed hypersensitivity reactions which would be deleterious to the mucosa as it is continuously exposed to food or airborne antigens.

All intestinal epithelial cells are derived from stem cells in the crypts. In the adult small intestine each crypt is a clonal unit harboring a ring of anchored stem cells near the crypt base that give rise to multiple cell types which migrate upward in columns onto several adjacent villi [15-17]. The epithelium of each villus is thus derived from several surrounding crypts. Paneth cells migrate to the bottom of the crypts, while the other cell types; goblet cells, absorptive enterocytes and enteroendocrine cells, migrate from the crypt proliferating compartment to the top of the villi where they eventually undergo apoptosis and are shed into the lumen [18]. The factors and signals that control proliferation and differentiation remain poorly characterized but mesenchymal cells in the underlying lamina propria and the basal lamina extracellular matrix components are known to play a crucial role in epithelial differentiation [19]. More recently, cell adhesion molecules such as the cadherins have been shown to control cell proliferation and differentiation [20].

Follicle-associated epithelium is dependent on the proliferation of cells located in the crypts surrounding the mucosal lymphoid follicles. The cells originate from the same ring of crypt stem cells which differentiate into absorptive enterocytes, goblet cells and enteroendocrine cells and migrate onto villi. Cells on the opposite wall of the same crypt move onto the dome where they acquire the features of M cells and distinct follicle-associated enterocytes [21]. As they emerge from the crypt, differentiating M cells begin endocytic activity, fail to assemble brush borders, and acquire intraepithelial lymphocytes and the characteristic pocket.

Antigen sampling in mucosal tissues

To obtain antigen samples, the immune system requires the collaboration of epithelial cells with antigen-presenting and lymphoid cells. The challenge faced by mucosal epithelial tissues is to transport antigen samples across these barriers without compromising their integrity and protective functions. In stratified epithelia, such as in the oral cavity and the vagina, motile antigen presenting cells, the Langerhans cells are able to migrate into the intraepithelial spaces, where they may obtain samples to carry back to local mucosal lymphoid tissues or distant lymph nodes [13, 22].

In the simple epithelium of the gut and airways where intercellular spaces are sealed by tight junctions, antigens cross the epithelial barrier by interacting with resident specialized epithelial M cells in the follicle-associated epithelium, that covers organized lymphoid tissues within the mucosa [1, 2] or with motile dendritic cells [23]. Thus, the fates of antigens and pathogens that cross epithelial barriers may differ, depending on the mucosal site: for example they may be released at M cell basolateral surfaces and taken up by intra- or subepithelial antigen-presenting cells in the dome region of o-MALT (organized mucosal associated lymphoid tissue) [24] or they may be carried by dendritic leukocytes to distant inductive sites as has been shown in the lower airways [25, 26]. Dendritic cells have also recently been identified in the colon [27], although it is not known whether they are able to migrate to the draining lymph nodes. These early events at mucosal surfaces may determine the immunological outcomes of antigen transport and the efficacy of mucosal vaccine strategies.

Plasticity of epithelial antigen sampling

Both resident (M cells) and migratory (Langerhans cells and dendritic cells) antigen sampling systems that are associated with simple or stratified epithelia are plastic and regulated by environmental and host factors. The microflora is able to influence the host cell differentiation programs, thereby creating favorable niches on the one hand and, on the other hand, affecting the host adaptive mucosal immune system. For instance, in germ free mice exposed to a single commensal organism, the number and the size of Peyer's patches rapidly increases [28].

There is indirect evidence that cell contacts and/or soluble factors from mucosal lymphoid follicles play an important role in induction of FAE and M cells. The fact that the follicle side of follicle-associated crypts shows distinct features including lack of Paneth cells, M cell-like glycosylation patterns and lack of polymeric immunoglobulin receptors, suggests that factors from o-MALT may act very early in the differentiation pathway, inducing crypt cells to commit to FAE phenotypes. On the other hand, factors or cells from the follicle or the lumen may also act later, to convert some of the FAE enterocyte-like cells to antigen-transporting M cells. Such a phenotypic conversion of enterocytes with the loss of digestive functions and the concomitant acquisition of translocation activity has recently been demonstrated in a reconstituted *in vitro* system. In this model differentiated human intestinal cells (Caco-2 cells) have been converted into cells that share many features of M cells by co-cultivating them with lymphocytes expressing B cell markers [29]. Several lines of evidence support a role for B cells as the major inductive partner. For example, we and others have analyzed Peyer's patch and FAE formation in immune-deficient mice and have found that whereas small Peyer's patches with typical M cells are found in nude mice lacking thymus-dependent T cells (unpublished observation) no Peyer's patches and M cells develop in mice devoid of B cells (Debard *et al.*, manuscript in preparation). The interaction of lymphoid cells, probably B cells, with the follicle-associated epithelium induces two types of changes: a general transcriptional down-regulation in all FAE epithelial cells of nutritional enzymes and membrane transporters, and more drastic changes restricted to M cells. The possibility of enterocyte-M cell conversion is supported by the observation that cells with both enterocyte and M cell features are present in FAE [30] and that M cell numbers are modified by short-term exposure to a non-intestinal bacterium inconventional rabbits [31]. As intestinal epithelial cells are known to release cytokines in response to bacterial invasion, one could therefore imagine that bacterial colonization or invasion of FAE enterocytes results in epithelial cell signal transduction events which influence underlying lymphoid cells, which in turn induce conversion of local enterocytes to the M cell phenotype. It is possible that this induction involves direct lymphocyte-epithelial cell contacts, including lymphocyte migration into the epithelium.

The importance of lymphoid cells in induction of the FAE is supported by the fact that injection of heterologous Peyer's patch cells into the submucosa of normal mice resulted in local assembly of a new lymphoid follicle and *de novo* appearance of FAE [29]. The three-way interaction of epithelium, microorganisms and lymphoid cells seen in the FAE provides a dramatic demonstration of the phenotypic plasticity of the intestinal epithelium.

Ontogeny of o-MALT

Appearance of FAE and M cells appears to follow the development of o-MALT. Development of organized lymphoid tissues seems to be constitutive with distinct frequencies and distribution depending on the species, with Peyer's patches appearing during the fetal life in the absence of exogenous antigenic stimulation [32]. For example, in humans Peyer's patches in the small intestine can be detected around 11 weeks of gestation [33]. In mice three distinct stages in Peyer's patch formation have recently been described [34]. First VCAM-1$^+$ stromal cell clusters appear at day 15.5. Two days later round cells expressing MHC class II, IL-7 receptors or CD4 accumulate and acquire T or B cell markers one day later. These aggregates are initially detected in the upper jejunum and extend to the colon as the number of clusters increases and, at birth, their number reaches up to eight or nine. Distinct mechanisms appear to control o-MALT ontogeny in the gut and probably elsewhere. At present, however, nothing is known about the underlying molecular and cellular events that determine where o-MALT sites will form, but it is likely that local secretion of chemokines, cytokines or other growth factors by stromal and epithelial cells recruit monocytes and lymphoid cells and control their tissue organization. This is supported by recent experiments in which the genes coding for cytokines, chemokines and their receptors have been deleted in mice.

Cytokines of the tumor necrosis factor (TNF) family play a role in the organogenesis of peripheral and mucosal lymphoid tissues. The development of peripheral lymph nodes and Peyer's patches has been analyzed in mice deficient in TNFα, lymphotoxins (LTα, LTβ), and their corresponding receptors (TNFR p55 and p75; LTβR). Disruption of TNFRp75 did not impair T cell function and the phenotypic abnormalities in lymphoid organs were minimal. The resistance of these mice to septic shock and TNF-induced death was increased [35]. In contrast, inactivation of LTα and LTβ genes caused severe lesions, with the total absence of Peyer's patches and peripheral lymph nodes, except mesenteric and cervical. In addition no primary or secondary B cell follicles were found in the spleen [36, 37].

Disruption of TNFα or TNFRp55 genes did not affect macroscopically lymph node and spleen organogenesis. Distinct T and B cell zones persisted but the organs lacked organized networks of follicular dendritic cells with no recognizable primary and secondary follicles [38, 39]. In contrast, Peyer's patches were markedly reduced in number organization with small and flat follicles containing few B cells. This suggests that TNF and TNFRp55 do not participate in primary organogenesis but are critically involved in the development of mature secondary structures [39].

References

1. Neutra MR, Frey A, Kraehenbuhl JP. Epithelial M cells: gateways for mucosal infection and immunization. *Cell* 1996; 86: 345-8.
2. Neutra MR, Kraehenbuhl JP. M cells as a pathway for antigen uptake and processing. In: Kagnoff M, Kiyono H, eds. *Essentials of Mucosal Immunology*. Academic Press, 1996: 29-36.
3. Bry L, Falk PG, Midtvedt T, Gordon JI. A model of host-microbial interactions in an open mammalian ecosystem. *Science* 1996; 273: 1380-3.
4. Colgan SP, Parkos CA, Delp C, Arnaout MA, Madara JL. Neutrophil migration across cultured intestinal epithelial monolayers is modulated by epithelial exposure to IFN-gamma in a highly polarized fashion. *J Cell Biol* 1993; 120: 785-98.
5. Eckmann L, Kagnoff MF, Fierer J. Intestinal epithelial cells as watchdogs for the natural immune system. *Trends Microbiol* 1995; 3: 118-20.

6. Kühn R, Löhler J, Rennick D, Rajewsky K, Müller W. Interleukin-10-deficient mice develop chronic enterocolitis. *Cell* 1993; 75: 263-74.
7. Sadlack B, Merz H, Schorle H, Schimpl A, Feller AC, Horak I. Ulcerative colitis-like disease in mice with a disrupted interleukin-2 gene. *Cell* 1993; 75: 253-61.
8. Neutra MR, Pringault E, Kraehenbuhl JP. Antigen sampling across epithelial barriers and induction of mucosal immune responses. *Annu Rev Immunol* 1996; 14: 275-300.
9. Guy-Grand D, Cuénod-Jabri B, Malassis-Seris M, Selz F, Vassalli P. Complexity of the mouse gut T cell immune system: identification of two distinct natural killer T cell intraepithelial lineages. *Eur J Immunol* 1996; 26: 2248-56.
10. Lefrançois L. Phenotypic complexity of intraepithelial lymphocytes of the small intestine. *J Immunol* 1991; 147: 1746-51.
11. Li Y, Yio XY, Mayer L. Human intestinal epithelial cell-induced $CD8^+$ T cell activation is mediated through CD8 and the activation of CD8-associated p56lck. *J Exp Med* 1995; 182: 1079-88.
12. Boismenu R, Feng L, Xia YY, Chang JC, Havran WL. Chemokine expression by intraepithelial gamma delta T cells. Implications for the recruitment of inflammatory cells to damaged epithelia. *J Immunol* 1996; 157: 985-92.
13. Eriksson K, Ahlfors E, George-Chandy A, Kaiserlian D, Czerkinsky C. Antigen presentation in the murine oral epithelium. *Immunology* 1996; 88: 147-52.
14. Panja A, Blumberg RS, Balk SP, Mayer L. CD1d is involved in T cell-intestinal epithelial cell interactions. *J Exp Med* 1993; 178: 1115-9.
15. Cheng H, Leblond CP. Origin, differentiation and renewal of the four main epithelial cell types in the mouse small intestine. *Am J Anat* 1974; 141: 461-80.
16. Schmidt GH, Wilkinson MM, Ponder BAJ. Cell migration pathway in the intestinal epithelium: an *in situ* marker system using mouse aggregation chimeras. *Cell* 1985; 40: 425-9.
17. Hermiston ML, Simon TC, Crossman MW, Gordon JI. Model systems for studying cell fate specification and differentiation in the gut epithelium. In: Johnson LR, Alpers DH, Christensen J, Jacobson ED, Walsh JH, eds. *Physiology of the Gastrointestinal Tract*. New York: Raven Press, 1994: 521-70.
18. Gravieli Y, Sherman Y, Ben-Sasson SA. Identification of programmed cell death *in situ via* specific labeling of nuclear DNA fragmentation. *J Cell Biol* 1992; 119: 493-501.
19. Simon-Assmann P, Kedinger M. Heterotypic cellular cooperation in gut morphogenesis and differentiation. Semin. *Cell Biol* 1993; 4: 221-30.
20. Hermiston ML, Wong MH, Gordon JI. Forced expression of e-cadherin in the mouse intestinal epithelium slows cell migration and provides evidence for nonautonomous regulation of cell fate in a self-renewing system. *Genes Dev* 1996; 10: 985-96.
21. Bye WA, Allan CH, Trier JS. Structure, distribution and origin of M cells in Peyer's patches of mouse Ileum. *Gastroenterology* 1984; 86: 789-801.
22. Miller CJ, McChesney M, Moore PF. Langerhans cells, macrophages and lymphocyte subsets in the cervix and vagina of rhesus macaques. *Lab Invest* 1992; 67: 628-34.
23. Nelson DJ, McMenamin C, McWilliam AS, Brenan M, Holt PG. Development of the airway intraepithelial dendritic cell network in the rat from class II major histocompatibility (Ia)-negative precursors: differential regulation of Ia expression at different levels of the respiratory tract. *J Exp Med* 1994; 179: 203-12.
24. Kelsall BL, Strober W. Dendritic cells of the gastrointestinal tract. *Springer Sem Immunopathol* 1997; 18: 409-20.
25. Holt PG. Pulmonary dendritic cell populations. *Advances in experimental medicine and biology*. New York, 1993; 329: 557-62.

26. McWilliam AS, Napoli S, Marsh AM, Pemper FL, Nelson DJ, Pimm CL, Stumbles PA, Wells TNC, Holt PG. Dendritic Cells Are Recruited Into the Airway Epithelium During the Inflammatory Response to a Broad Spectrum of Stimuli. *J Exp Med* 1996; 184: 2429-32.
27. Maric I, Holt PG, Perdue MH, Bienenstock J. Class II MHC antigen (la)-bearing dendritic cells in the epithelium of the rat intestine. *Immunology* 1996; 156: 1408-14.
28. Shroff KE, Meslin K, Cebra JJ. Commensal enteric bacteria engender a self-limiting humoral mucosal immune response while permanently colonizing the gut. *Infect Immun* 1995; 63: 3904-13.
29. Kernéis S, Bogdanova A, Kraehenbuhl JP, Pringault E. Conversion by Peyer's patch lymphocytes of human enterocytes into M cells that transport bacteria. *Science* 1997; 277: 948-52.
30. Savidge TC. The life and times of an intestinal M cell. *Trends Microbiol* 1996; 4: 301-6.
31. Borghesi C, Regoli M, Bertelli E, Nicoletti C. Modifications of the follicle-associated epithelium by short-term exposure to a non-intestinal bacterium. *J Pathol* 1996; 180: 326-32.
32. Griebel PJ, Hein WR. Expanding the role of Peyer's patches in B-cell ontogeny. *Immunol Today* 1996; 17: 30-9.
33. Spencer J, MacDonald TT, Finn T, Isaacson PG. The development of gut-associated lymphoid tissue in the terminal ileum of fetal human intestine. *Clinical and experimental immunology*. Oxford, 1986; 64: 536-43.
34. Adachi S, Yoshida H, Kataoka H, Nishikawa S. Three distinctive steps in Peyer patch formation of murine embryo. *Int Immunol* 1997; 9: 507-14.
35. Erickson SL, de Sauvage FJ, Kikly K, Carver-Moore K, Pitts-Meek S, Gillett N, Sheehan KC, Schreiber RD, Goeddel DV, Moore MW. Decreased sensitivity to tumour-necrosis factor but normal T cell development in TNF receptor-2-deficient mice. *Nature* 1994; 372: 560-3.
36. Alimzhanov MB, Kuprash DV, Koscovilbois MH, Luz A, Turetskaya RL, Tarakhovsky A, Rajewsky K, Nedospasov SA, Pfeffer K. Abnormal Development of Secondary Lymphoid Tissues in Lymphotoxin Beta-Deficient Mice. *Proc Natl Acad Sci USA* 1997; 94: 9302-7.
37. De Togni P, Goellner J, Ruddle NH, Streeter PR, Fick A, Mariathasan S, Smith SC, Carlson R, Shornick LP, Strauss-Schoenberger J, Russell JH, Karr R, Chaplin DD. Abnormal development of peripheral lymphoid organs in mice deficient in lymphotoxin. *Science* 1994; 264: 703-6.
38. Neumann B, Machleidt T, Lifka A, Pfeffer K, Vestweber D, Mak TW, Holzmann B, Kronke M. Crucial role of 55-kilodalton TNF receptor in TNF-induced adhesion molecule expression and leukocyte organ infiltration. *J Immunol* 1996; 156: 1587-93.
39. Pasparakis M, Alexopoulou L, Episkopou V, Kollias G. Immune and inflammatory responses in TNF-alpha-deficient mice – a critical requirement for TNF-alpha in the formation of primary B cell follicles, follicular dendritic cell networks and germinal centers, and in the maturation of the humoral immune response. *J Exp Med* 1996; 184: 1397-411.

Recent advances in the pathogenesis of gastrointestinal bacterial infections.
P. Rampal, P. Boquet, eds. John Libbey Eurotext, Paris © 1998, pp. 65-79.

Bacterial adherence, transmembrane signaling and epithelial cytokine responses

Maria Hedlund[1], Majlis Svensson[1], Long Hang[1], Hugh Connell[1], Björn Wullr[2], Gabriela Godaly[1], Gisela Otto[3], Masashi Haraoka[1], Björn Frendéus[1], Catharina Svanborg[1]

Departments of [1] Medical Microbiology (Division of Clinical Immunology), [2] Urology, [3] Department of Infectious Diseases; Lund University, Lund, Sweden

Mucosal pathogens evoke an acute inflammatory response. The severity of infection reflects the magnitude of this response. Local symptoms result from inflammation at the site of infection and systemic symptoms are caused by the spread of inflammatory mediators [1-3], bacteria or bacterial components to distant tissues that respond to these signals. In contrast to pathogens, members of the indigenous microflora do not seem to trigger inflammation at the local site of infection. It is the response to the bacteria, not the pathogens *per se* that cause most of the tissue pathology.

According to the traditional view, mucosal immune mechanisms have evolved to keep the integrity of the mucosal barrier and prevent entry of microbes and macromolecules. IgA antibodies prevent attachment, and secreted antimicrobial effectors like defensins prevent the microbes from reaching the tissues alive. Inflammation has always been considered as a disruptive force, responsible for asthma, inflammatory bowel disease, ulcers or interstitial cystitis. More recently it has become evident that celles in mucosal surfaces communicate quite actively with invading microbes, and that mucosal inflammation is crucial for the antimicrobial defense.

We study two aspects of mucosal inflammation; the molecular mechanisms by which bacteria trigger the first cellular response at mucosal sites, and the consequences of that response for resistance to infection. While different mucosal pathogens have evolved highly specialized mechanisms to localize to their site of infection in the human host, and to trigger inflammation at these sites, the overall strategies are quite similar. This chapter will describe host microbe interactions based on results from the *E. coli* urinary tract infection model. The pathogenesis may be summarized as follows.

1. The uropathogenic *E. coli* strains become established at mucosal sites outside the urinary tract; usually the colon and/or the outer genital area. It is likely that many of the virulence associated traits of uropathogenic *E. coli* have evolved to adapt them to colonization of the large intestine, and not to facilitate invasion of

the urinary tract. For example, the same adherence factors that later promote disease in the kidneys enhance persistence in the colonic flora. Like many other bacterial pathogens, the uropathogenic strains reside at one mucosal site and, by accident show enhanced fitness for a second site (lungs, ear, meninges, kidneys).
2. The uropathogens ascend into the urinary tract and establish numbers of 10^5 cfu/ml or more. Those that express P fimbriae and other adhesins are thought to have a considerable advantage during this phase. Adherence is thought to allow bacteria to persist, especially in patients with normal bladder function. Antibacterial peptides and the other hostile constituents of the urine contribute to resistance during this phase, but the details are poorly understood.
3. Bacteria make contact with epithelial cells lining the urinary tract and start the acute inflammatory response. The magnitude of this response and the site within the urinary tract determine disease severity. Kidney infections result in both local and systemic inflammation, and acute pyelonephritis can be a life threatening condition. Acute cystitis is characterized by acute inflammation localized to the bladder. Attachment shows a clear-cut association to disease severity in human patients and in animal models. Mutational inactivation of adhesion dramatically reduces bacterial persistence and inflammation.
4. In about 30% of patients with acute pyelonephritis, bacteria cross the mucosal barrier and invade the blood stream, causing urosepsis. P fimbriae mediated adherence and hemolysin production have been implicated in this process.
5. Bacteria are cleared from the tissues through the action of innate immune mechanisms, especially polymorphonuclear phagocytes. Bacteria counteract these effectors of inflammation by production of LPS, capsular polysaccharides and aerobactin.

Epithelial cells are the primary targets for attaching bacteria

Epithelial cells form the mucosal barrier and are a logical first target for microbial attack. Mucosal pathogens attach to the epithelial cells through highly specific mechanisms. Fimbriae-associated surface lectins bind to oligosaccharide receptor sequences in cell surface glycoconjugates [4]. Uropathogenic *E. coli* express type 1 fimbriae, recognizing mannosylated glycoproteins, S fimbriae recognizing Sialic acid residues on glycoproteins and Dr fimbriae recognizing receptors with Dr blood group specificity.

Early epidemiological studies showed disease severity to be associated with one specific adhesive interaction; that of P-fimbriae binding to the globoseries of glycolipids [4-6]. Subsequent studies in animal models showed that P-fimbriae negative mutants have reduced ability to survive in the urinary tract and to cause inflammation [7-11].

The receptors for *E. coli* P-fimbriae are Galα1-4Galβ-containing oligosaccharide sequences bound to ceramide in the globoseries of glycolipids [4, 12]. These glycolipids occur in urinary tract epithelial cells and in kidney tissue [4, 13]. Individual variation in receptor expression influences the susceptibility to infection with P-fimbriated *E. coli* [14].

The receptor binding domain of the fimbriae resides in the G adhesin at the tip of the fimbriae, and is encoded by the papG sequences [15]. The *pa*pG adhesin variants recognize different Galα1-4Galβ-oligosaccharide isoreceptors [16-19], and differ in disease association [16, 20, 21]. The mechanisms underlying these differences have not been clarified, but they may relate to the propensity of the P-fimbriated strains to induce a mucosal and systemic inflammatory response.

Epithelial cytokine responses

According to the conventional wisdom, inflammation is handled by specialized inflammatory cells like macrophages, neutrophils and mast cells. In order for a mucosal pathogen to reach and activate those cells it would have to pass the mucosal barrier by invasion or to export proinflammatory products that reach the inflammatory cells.

In 1989 we first showed that epithelial cells can produce cytokines, and that bacteria stimulate a cytokine response in those cells. This observation altered our focus from the specialized inflammatory cells to stromal cells in the mucosal lining, and provided a framework to study epithelial cell attachment not just as a colonization mechanism, but as a key event in activation of mucusal inflammation.

Bacterial adherence enhances epithelial cell cytokine responses

The initial study of epithelial responses to bacteria used epithelial cell lines from the urinary tract [3]. Epithelial cell cytokine mRNA levels increased after bacterial stimulation as did the intracellular cytokine content and the secretion of cytokines. The cytokine repertoire differed between uroepithelial cells and non-epithelial cells like macrophages. Immunohistochemistry of human biopsies showed that the cells constitutively produced IL-8 and TGF-β, and that the IL-6 and IL-1 levels increased in response to infection. Immunoregulatory cytokines like IL-4, γ-IFN or IL-2 were not detected in epithelial cells, and there was no TNF.

Bacterial adherence was shown to enhance the epithelial cells cytokine response to *E. coli*. The evidence may be summarized as follows:

1. P-fimbriated and type 1-fimbriated *E. coli* strains elicited higher cytokine responses than isogenic, non-fimbriated strains [22-24].

2. Isolated P-fimbriae elicited epithelial cell cytokine responses. The activation required a functionally active G adhesin; fimbriae lacking the receptor-binding domain did not elicit a cytokine response [25].

3. Inhibition of epithelial cells glycolipid expression reduced both the adherence and the cytokine response to P-fimbriated *E. coli*, but had no effect on the cytokine response to type 1-fimbriated *E. coli*, that bind other glycoconjugate receptors [24].

4. Receptor analogues (globotetraosylceramide for P-fimbriae and α-methyl-D-mannoside for type 1-fimbriae) inhibited bacterial adherence and epithelial cell cytokine responses [9-23].

These observations suggested that fimbriae-receptor interactions activate epithelial cell cytokine responses, and that the receptor specificity of the fimbriae helps direct these responses.

P-fimbriae and the ceramide signaling pathway

The host cell receptors for P-fimbriae are the globoseries of glycosphingolipids [4]. These neutral glycosphingolipids consists of Galα1-4Galβ-containing oligosaccharide sequences of varying chain length bound to ceramide in the outer leaflet of the lipid bilayer of mammalian cells. Ceramide has been shown to act as a second messenger in cell signaling and to activate downstream pathways involved in apoptosis and other cellular responses [26-28]. We recently demonstrated that P fimbriated *E. coli* activate the ceramide signaling patway in a human kidney cell line [29]. The concentration of free ceramide and ceramide 1-phosphate increased to reach a peak around 20 min after the onset of stimulation with P fimbriated bacteria. In contrast, there was no increase in ceramide levels in cells exposed to recombinant type 1 fimbriated bacteria or to the vector control.

Ceramide signaling is known to involve Ser/Thr specific protein kinases [30]. Inhibitors of Ser/Thr kinases were shown to block the P-fimbriae induced cytokine response, but had no effect on the IL-6 response to type 1 fimbriated strains. Tyrosine kinase inhibitors, in contrast, reduced the cytokine response to type 1 fimbriated but not to P fimbriated bacteria. These results show that:

1) P-fimbriated *E. coli* activate the ceramide signaling pathway, which contributes to the cytokine response to these bacteria in human kidney cells.

2) Type 1 fimbriae induce a cytokine response through different transmembrane signaling events.

3) Enhancement of cell activation by fimbriae is not simply due to the approximation of other bacterial factors to the cell surface; it is directly influenced by the receptor specificity of the fimbriae.

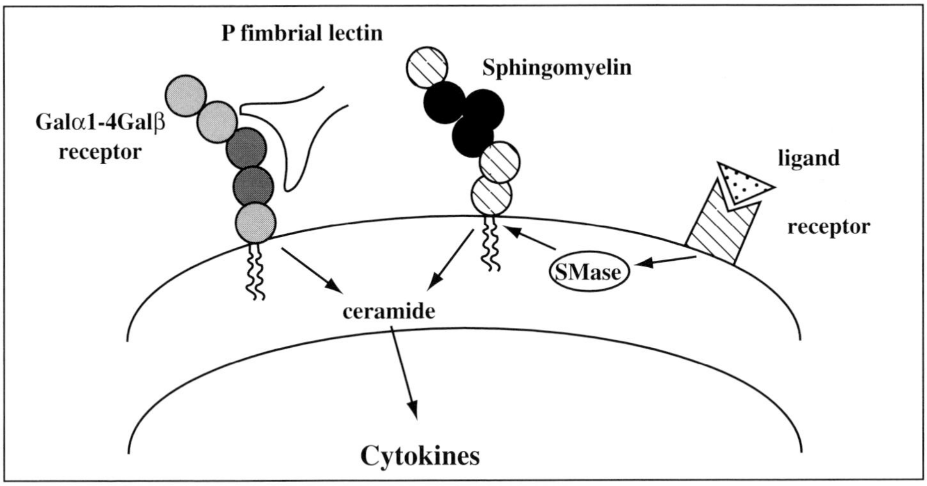

Figure 1. The ceramide signaling pathway. a) Ligands like FAS, IL-1α and TNF bind their respective cell surface receptor, and activate endogenous sphingomyelinases that release ceramide. Down-stream activation includes upregulation of NF-κB and may lead to cytokine production by the activated cells. b) Mechanisms by which P-fimbriated *E. coli* might activate the ceramide signaling pathway. P-fimbriated *E. coli* do not release ceramide from sphingomyelin, but rather from the receptor glycolipids. P-fimbriae recognizes the oligosaccharide portion of the globoseries of glycolipids and cause the release of ceramide from this molecule.

Molecular sources of ceramide

Ceramide is not released from sphingomyelin

Ceramide is the membrane anchoring domain of sphingomyelin, gangliosides and neutral glycosphingolipids. Agonists like TNFα, IL-1β and FAS bind to cell surfaces *via* their respective receptors and activate sphingomyelinases that cleave sphingomyelin to release ceramide [31-34]. We have shown that ceramide of this origin can activate cytokine responses in our *in vitro* system. Exogenous sphingomyelinase, TNFα and IL-1β that cleave sphingomyelin, release ceramide and stimulated IL-6 production in the A498 cells. P fimbriated *E. coli* did not cause detectable breakdown of sphingomyelin in those cells. Bacteria did not produce sphingomyelinases and the levels of endogenous acid or neutral sphingomyelinases in the cells were low. These results suggested that the release of ceramide following *E. coli* infection is not from sphingomyelin.

Is ceramide derived from the globoseries of glycosphingolipids?

The possible release of ceramide from the receptor glycolipids in *E. coli* stimulated cells was studied. Galactose containing glycosphingolipids were prelabeled with radioactive galactose. The loss of galactose label accompanying ceramide release was examined in glycosphingolipid extracts from cells obtained at various times after stimulation with P fimbriated *E. coli*. The amount of Galα1-4Galβ glycosphingolipid in the tri-, tetra-, and penta- to okta-saccharide region was quantitated by TLC and autoradiography. A significant reduction in the total lipid bound radioactive galactose was detected in cells exposed to P fimbriated *E. coli* compared to unstimulated control cells. These findings are consistent with an effect of P fimbriated *E. coli* on their receptor glycolipids.

LPS is not a costimulatory factor

Endotoxin (lipopolysaccharide, LPS) is an integral component of the outer membrane of Gram negative bacteria. Release of LPS in the circulation activates neutrophil, monocyte and macrophage inflammatory responses. The interaction of LPS with monocytes results in the release of pro-inflammatory cytokines such as TNF, IL-6 and IL-1. The endotoxic activity resides in the lipid A portion of the molecule. Alterations in lipid A may change the biologic activity of LPS. For example, LPS from *E. coli* strains expressing non-myristoylated lipid A failed to activate monocytes and endothelial cells [35].

Cell activation requires recognition of LPS at the cell surface and induction of transmembrane signaling. Several surface proteins have been shown to be involved in the initiation of a secretory response after recognition of LPS. Binding of LPS to the serum protein LBP enhances cell activation through membrane bound CD14, but CD14 is attached to the cell membrane only by a glucosylphosphatidyl inositol anchor, which suggest additional signal transduction molecules. The LPS responsiveness in cells like endothelial cells, which lack surface bound CD14, can be reconstituted by addition of serum which contain soluble CD14.

Is there a role for bacterial endotoxin in epithelial cytokine production and is LPS acting in synergy with fimbriae induced ceramide signaling. LPS is a structural analogue of ceramide, and has been suggested to bypass ceramide as an activator of Ser/Thr specific signaling mechanisms [36]. This effect was found in CD14 positive cells and in the presence of LBP. Synergy between LPS and fimbriae has been observed in the urinary tract of mice [37]. P-fimbriae carry LPS as an integral part of the adhesin and could thereby function as LPS presenters by approximating the LPS molecule to the host cell surface.

We have studied LPS as a co-signal or second signal in P-fimbriae induced cytokine responses. The results suggest that LPS is not required for cell activation.

1. A498 kidney epithelial cells are refractory to purified LPS and a concentration of 100 μg/ml is required in order to activate cytokine production. Differences in the LPS polysaccharide structure do not influence the poor response.

2. The epithelial cells do not express surface CD14 as shown by immunochemistry with monoclonal anti-CD14 antibodies. Both the A498 cell line and human biopsies were examined. Stimulation with LPS or whole bacteria could not induce CD14

expression or CD14 mRNA production. Addition of soluble CD14 could not reconstitute the LPS responsiveness of the A498 cells.

3. LPS inhibitors like BPI and PolymyxinB did not affect epithelial cytokine responses to whole bacteria.

4. *E. coli* strains expressing non-myristoylated LPS were transformed with sequences encoding the P-fimbriae. The cytokine response to P fimbriated isogens in normal or dysfunctional LPS backgrounds were compared. The transformant expressing dysfunctional LPS induced a higher cytokine response than strains expressing normal LPS. This suggested that LPS, rather than contributing to the cytokine response, interfered with cell activation.

Do P fimbriated *E. coli* invade uroepithelial cells?

The *E. coli* strains that cause urosepsis pass from the local site of infection in the urinary tract, across the epithelial barrier and into the bloodstream [38-40]. The mechanisms have been examined *in vitro* in the transwell model with bacteria added to the upper well of confluent uroepithelial layers and the numbers reaching the lower well calculated at various times after infection. Marked virulence-related differences in bacterial translocation across uroepithelial cell layers were observed. Urosepsis and pyelonephritis isolates crossed the cell layers soon after infection of the upper well. *E. coli* HB101, used as a host for recombinant plasmids, did not pass the cell layer. The P fimbriated recombinant strains formed an intermediary group. They passed the cell layer more efficiently than *E. coli* HB101, but did not reach numbers comparable to the disease isolates unless a very high inoculum concentration was used. The results demonstrate that P-fimbriae enhance epithelial transmigration but that additional virulence factors are needed to reach the efficiency of the disease isolates.

The effect of P-fimbriae on bacterial transmigration varied with the G adhesin class. The *pap*G encoded P fimbrial adhesins differ in isoreceptor specificity and in disease association [17-21, 42, 43]. The *pap*GAD110 or *pap*GIA12 adhesin sequences predominate in acute pyelonephritis and in blood isolates from patient with urosepsis [21, 44]. The phenotype, described as the class II P fimbrial adhesin, binds to the whole family of Galα1-4Galβ containing glycoconjugates, with a possible preference for globotetraosylceramide or longer chain globoseries of glycosphingolipids [18]. The *pap*GJ96 adhesin (class I) is expressed by members of a single clone, and is extremely rare in most clinical UTI materials [21, 45]. The adhesin recognizes terminal Galα1-4Galβ residues, preferentially in globotriaocylceramide. The *prs*GJ96 adhesin (class III), occurs at a fairly low frequency (10-30%) in UTI isolates with some overrepresentation in acute cystitis [21]. The adhesin recognizes a terminal GalNAc-α-linked to a globoserie core [18]. The *prs*GJ96 expressing strains preferentially infect individuals of blood group A [18]. In this study, the P fimbriated recombinant strains expressing class II G-adhesins passed uroepithelial cell monolayers more efficiently than the transformants expressing the *pap*GJ96 or *prs*GJ96 adhesins. These results are consistent with the disease association of this class of P-fimbriae.

The disease isolates, and to a lesser extent the P fimbriated recombinants, disrupted intercellular junctions, caused rounding up of the cells and detachment from the filters. Infection-induced detachment of the epithelial cells, has previously been observed *in vivo* in urinary tract infection models. Aronson *et al.* showed that certain uropathogenic *E. coli* strains caused epithelial shedding when introduced into the urinary tract and that the shedding depended on the host background, since there was a difference between C3H/HeN LPS responder and C3H/HeJ LPS non responder mice [46]. Detachment was, however, not due to direct bacterial toxicity for the A498 cells, since there was no reduction in the viability of infected cells during the experimental time period, as determined by trypan blue exclusion. Preliminary results suggest that the cells undergo apoptosis, but only later in the infection process (Svensson *et al.* in preparation).

Studies on intestinal epithelial cells have suggested that invasion is required in order to trigger a cytokine-response [47, 48]. Since we found no evidence for bacterial invasion under the conditions that caused cell activation, intracellular infection did not appear to be required for activation of a uroepithelial cell cytokine response.

Fimbriae, chemokine responses and neutrophil migration across infected epithelial cell layers

The epithelial cytokine response provides a first signal of local inflammation. Subsequently, non-epithelial cells may be recruited or activated by the epithelial cells and a local network is formed. The release of chemokines stimulates the migration of inflammatory cells like neutrophils to the urinary tract. The last part of this process may be studied *in vitro* using the transwell model. In this model, *E. coli* stimulate neutrophil migration across human uroepithelial cell layers [23]. We investigated the role of the neutrophil chemokine interleukin-8 (IL-8) in this process [49, 50]. *E. coli* and IL-1α stimulated urinary tract epithelial layers to secrete IL-8 and induced transepithelial neutrophil migration. Anti-IL-8 antibody reduced neutrophil migration across epithelial cell layers to background levels indicating a central role for this chemokine in the migration process. Furthermore addition of recombinant IL-8 to unstimulated cell layers was sufficient to induce migration. The IL-8 dependence of neutrophil migration was maintained after removal of soluble IL-8 by washing of the cell layers. Flow cytometry analysis with FITC-IL-8 confirmed IL-8's ability to bind to the epithelial cell surface. Indirect immunofluorescence using confocal laser scanning microscopy showed IL-8 receptor A reduced neutrophil migration, but anti-IL-8 associated with the epithelial cell layers. Prior incubation of neutrophils with antibodies to the IL-8 receptor B antibody had no effect on neutrophil migration. These results demonstrate that IL-8 plays a key role in *E. coli* or IL-1α induced transuroepithelial migration, and suggest that epithelial cells IL-8 interacts with IL-8RA on the neutrophil surface [50].

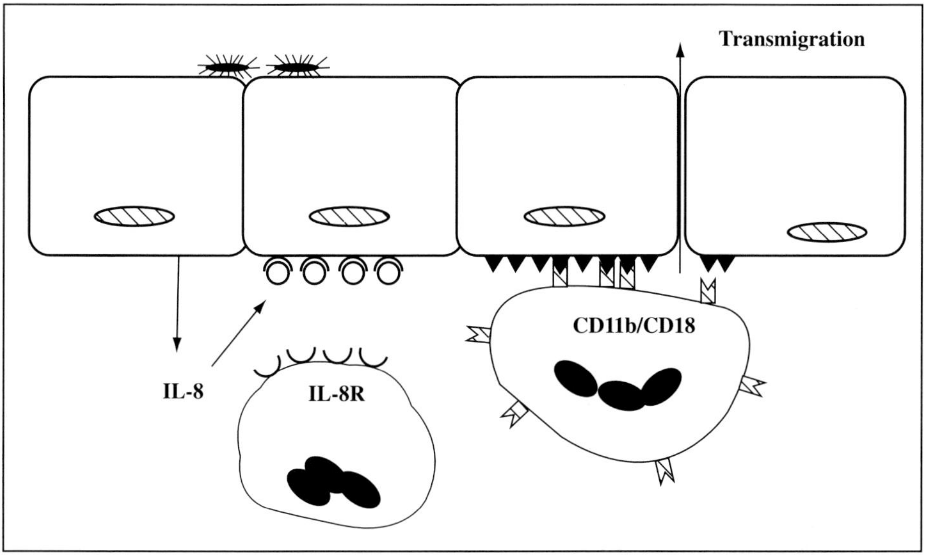

Figure 2. Bacteria enhance neutrophil migration across epithelial cell layers. a) Fimbriated bacteria upregulate cytokine expression, including C-X-C chemokines like IL-8. They also stimulate the expression of IL-8 receptors, resulting in an increase in surface-bound IL-8. Neutrophils bind *via* their IL-8 receptors. b) Bacteria stimulate the expression of cell-adhesion molecules (ICAM-1). Neutrophils bind *via* the CD11b/CD18 ligand.

The role of P and type 1 fimbriae for neutrophil migration was examined *in vitro* for *E. coli* infected uroepithelial cell layers and *in vivo* for recruitment into the infected mouse urinary tract [51]. Recombinant *E. coli* K-12 strains differing in P or type 1 fimbrial expression were used to infect confluent epithelial layers on the underside of transwell inserts. Neutrophils were added to the upper well, and their passage across the epithelial cell layers was quantitated. Infection with the P and type 1 fimbriated recombinant *E. coli* strains stimulated neutrophil migration to the same extent as a fully virulent clinical *E. coli* isolate, but the isogenic non-fimbriated vector control strains had no stimulatory effect. The enhancement of neutrophil migration was adhesion dependent; it was inhibited by soluble receptor analogues blocking the binding of P-fimbriae to the globoseries of glycosphingolipids or of type 1 fimbriae to mannosylated glycoprotein receptors. P and type 1 fimbriated *E. coli* triggered higher IL-8 secretion, and expression of functional IL-8 receptors than non-fimbriated controls, and the increase in neutrophil migration across infected cell layers was inhibited by anti-IL-8 antibodies. In a mouse infection model, P or type 1 fimbriated *E. coli* stimulated higher chemokine (MIP-2) and neutrophil responses than the non-fimbriated vector controls. The results demonstrated that transformation with the *pap* or *fim* DNA sequences is sufficient to convert an *E. coli* K-12 strain to a host response inducer, and that fimbriation enhances neutrophil recruitment *in vitro* and *in vivo*. Epithelial chemokine production provides a molecular link between the fimbriated bacteria that adhere to epithelial cells and tissue inflammation.

Fimbriae enhance the inflammatory response in the human urinary tract

The influence of bacterial adherence on the mucosal cytokine response has been examined in the human urinary tract. Intravesical inoculations with non-virulent bacteria were performed in an attempt to protect special patient groups against recurrent, symptomatic infections of the urinary tract. This strategy was based on clinical observations in children and adults with asymptomatic bacteriuria [52-54]. Those who were left untreated were shown to have a lower frequency of symptomatic recurrences than the patients who were given antibiotics in order to eliminate the bacteriuria. Follow up of the bacteriuria in the patients did not reveal adverse effects on renal function. This suggested that bacteriuria with a non-virulent strain could protect against infection with a more deleterious bacteria.

Patients with recurrent episodes of acute pyelonephritis due to neurogenic bladder disorders were enrolled in the colonization study. The role of bacterial adherence for the human urinary tract cytokine responses was studied using isogenic *E. coli* strains that differ in the expression of fimbriae. The patients were injected intravesically with *E. coli* 83972, and P fimbriated derivatives of this strain. *E. coli* 83972 pap_{IA2} had received the type of pap_{IA2} DNA sequences in the single-copy plasmid pREG153. The pap_{IA2} type of P-fimbriae has been shown to predominate among uropathogenic *E. coli* that cause acute pyelonephritis [21]. *E. coli* 83972 was selected for these studies due to its documented ability to persist in the human urinary tract [55]. It was originally isolated from a young girl with asymptomatic bacteriuria, who had carried it for three years without symptoms or adverse effects. The strain lacked the virulence traits that characterize acute pyelonephritis strains, and had been shown to colonize several human hosts without causing symptoms [55].

In order to examine the role of P-fimbriae for the induction of mucosal inflammation in the urinary tract isogenic *E. coli* strains differing in P fimbrial expression were deposited into the urinary bladder of human patients. The establishment of bacteriuria was recorded, and the persistence over time controlled using genetic markers. *In vivo* fimbrial expression was examined on cells harvested from urine without subculture, and the *pap* genotype was determined on subcultured organisms by DNA hybridization. The inflammatory ressponse was quantitated as neutrophil recruitment and cytokine secretion into the urine. The results demonstrated that P-fimbriae enhance the inflammatory response to infection. The evidence may be summarized as follows: The P fimbriated isogens expressing the $papG_{IA}$ and $prsG_{396}$ adhesins invariably caused higher neutrophil and cytokine responses than the non-fimbriated isogen. This effect was observed when all colonization events with the P-fimbriae positive and negative strains were compared in the patient group as a whole, and in individual patients colonized sequentially with P-fimbriae positive and negative isogens. Finally, cytokine responses varied with fimbrial expression during colonization of individual patients. Loss of fimbrial expression by the $papG_{IA2}$ positive isogen was accompanied by a reduction to background levels of the neutrophil, IL-6 and IL-8 responses. These results demonstrate that fimbriae-mediated adhrence enhances the virulence of uropathogenic *E. coli* through an effect on inflammation.

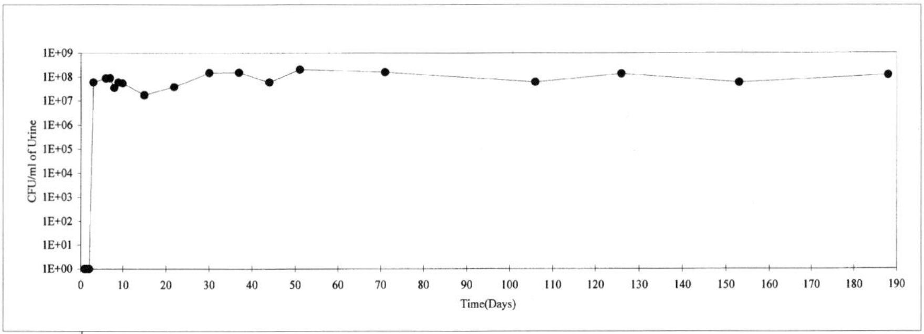

PMNs	1	4	1	4	3	0	1	8	1	0	0	0	8
IL-6	<15	<15	<15	<15	<15	<15	<15	<15	<15	<15	<15	<15	<15
IL-8	2.4	1.3	0.5	0.8	<0.031	0.2	1.2	0.8	1.1	1.6	1.1	0.4	1.2
1 kb plasmid		+				+	+		+	+	+	+	+
pap		+				+	+		–	–	–	–	–
HA	–	–	–	–	–	–	–	–	–	–	–	–	–

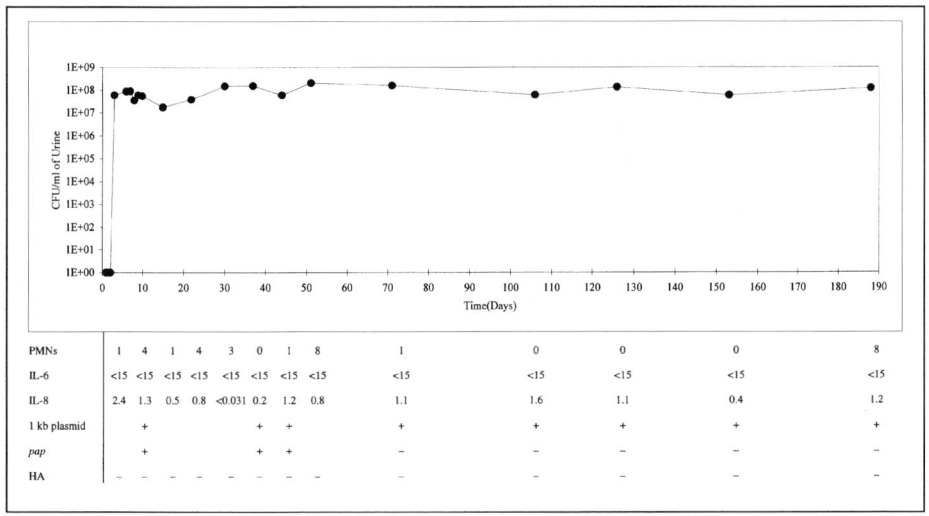

Figure 3. Longterm bacteriuria is established after intravesical inoculation with *E. coli* 83972 pap_{IA2}. The *pap* sequences are reatined but fimbrial expression is switched off in the urinary tract.

Cytokine responses and disease severity

Interleukin-6 responses were analyzed in serum and urine of 81 patients with febrile urinary tract infections (UTI) with (n = 24) or without (n = 57) bacteremia. All patients showed an IL-6 response in urine and/or serum. Bacteremic patients had higher serum IL-6 at inclusion and throughout the first 24 hours, and higher urine IL-6 from 6 hours after start of therapy than non-bacteremic patients. The kinetics of the IL-6 responses differed between the groups, with prolonged elevation of IL-6 in serum and urine in the bacteremic group. Patients with clinical signs of pyelonephritis had higher serum and urine IL-6 concentrations, and IL-6 high responders had higher temperature and CRP levels than low responders. The results demonstrate that IL-6 responses accompanyall cases of febrile UTI, and that themagnitude of the response reflects the disease severity. IL-6 in the circulation is not only generated by invading bacteria, but by spread of cytokines from the local site of infection. IL-6 from the urinary tract helps trigger the systemic host response, in both bacteremic and non-bacteremic febril UTI [56].

Inflammation and resistance to infection

It is generally believed that neutrophils are essential for bacterial clearance from the lungs, the brain and other tissues during systemic infection [57-59]. The mechanisms of microbial killing during the early stage of infection at mucosal sites are less well understood. Specific immunity including secretary IgA antibodies may be highly protective, but dysfunction's in specific immunity do not automatically increase the susceptibility to mucosal pathogens. Defects that impair the acute inflammatory response have, on the other hand, been shown to greatly impair bacterial clearance from mucosal sites, and to render mice highly susceptibility to Gram negative bacteria like *Salmonella, Escherichia coli* and *Haemophilus influenzae* [57-61]. Numerous indirect observations suggest that recruited neutrophils are important local effectors of the antibacterial host response [62, 63] but their role for resistance to mucosal infection has not been defined.

Neutrophil recruitment to mucosal sites requires a chemotactic gradient and expression of cell adhesion molecules by the epithelial cells. The neutrophils leave the blood stream, migrate to and cross the epithelial barrier into the lumen. Bacteria stimulate epithelial cells to secrete C-C as well as C-X-C chemokines [23, 47] and upregulate the epithelial cell expression of ICAM-1 [60]. Antibodies to IL-8, ICAM-1 and CD-11b have been shown to block neutrophil migration across *E. Coli* stimulated epithelial cell layers *in vitro* [49, 50]. These insights into the molecular mechanisms of neutrophil migration *in vitro* make it possible to interfere with neutrophil recruitment to mucosal sites *in vivo*, and to study the effects on bacterial infection.

We have characterized the chemokine response to *Escherichia coli* urinary tract infection, blocked neutrophil migratiçon with antibodies to neutrophil surface markers or chemokines, and examined the effect of peripheral neutrophil depletion on bacterial clearance. Intravesical infection with *E. coli* 1177, a fully virulent clinical isolate, triggered local production of C-C and C-X-C chemokines and stimulated neutrophil migration into the tissues and the urine. MIP-2 showed the most clear-cut correlation to urine neutrophil numbers and pretreatment of the mice with anti-MIP-2 inhibited neutrophil influx into the urine.

The peripheral neutrophil recruitment was abrogated using the granulocyte-specific monoclonal antibody RB6-8C5. There were no neutrophils in kidneys or bladders, and bacterial clearance from kidneys and bladders was drastically impaired. The results demonstrated that neutrophils are essential for bacterial clearance from the urinary tract. In contrast the anti-MIP-2 treated mice remained fully resistant to infection. The difference was explained using immunohistochemistry. Neutrophils were present in the kidneys of anti-MIP-2 treated mice but were unable to traverse the urothelium. MIP-2 was involved in neutrophil migration across the urothelium into the urine, but not in neutrophil recruitment from the circulation to the kidney tissue. Complex chemokine responses are required for neutrophil recruitment to infected mucosal sites.

Acknowledgements

These studies were supported by: the Swedish Medical Research Council; the Medical Faculty, University of Lund; the Swedish Medical Society; the Royal Physiographical Society of Lund; and the Österlund, the Crafoord, and Lundberg Foundations.

Summary

Mucosal pathogens trigger an acute inflammatory response. Epithelial cells and other mucosal cells respond to the presence of bacteria in highly specific ways, depending on the molecular interactions with the pathogen. The first wave of inflammatory mediators in the mucosal compartment sets up a network of interactions with local and recruited cells. The inflammatory cascade is amplified, and symptoms arise from the local and systemic release of the proinflammatory mediators.
The inflammatory response also includes effectors with antibacterial activity. Neutrophil cells are one example. They are essential for the elimination of bacteria from the mucosal tissues. This illustrates how inflammation is a double edged sword, essential for the acute pathology but also for resistance to infection.

References

1. De Man P, Jodal U, Lincoln K, Svanborg-Edén C. *J Infect Dis* 1998; 158: 29-35.
2. De Man P, van Kooten C, Arden L, Engberg I, Linder H, Svanborg-Edén C. *Infect Immun* 1989; 57: 3383-8.
3. Hedges S, Stenquist K, Lidin-Janson G, Martinell J, Sandberg T, Svanborg C. *J Infect Dis* 1992; 166: 653-6.
4. Leffler H, Svanborg-Edén C. *FEMS Microbiol Lett* 1980; 8: 127-34.
5. Leffler H, Svanborg-Edén C. *Infect Immun* 1981; 34: 920-9.
6. Väisänen R, Elo J, Tallgren L, Siitonen A, Mäkelä P, Svanborg-Edén C, Källenius G, Svenson S, Hultberg H, Korhonen T. *Lancet* 1981; Ii: 1366-9.
7. Hagberg L, Hull E, Hull S, Falkow S, Freter R, Svanborg-Edén C. *Infect Immun* 1983; 40: 265-72.
8. Svanborg-Edén C, Hagberg L, Leffler H, Lomberg H. In *The pathogenesis of Urinary Tract Infection. Infection* 1982; 10: 327-32.
9. Linder H, Engberg I, Hoschützky H, Mattsby Baltzer I, Svanborg-Edén C. *Infect Immun* 1991; 59: 4357-62.
10. Roberts J, Marklund BI, Ilver D, Haslam M, Kaak G, Baskin G, Möllby R, Winberg J, Normark S. *Proc Natl Acad Sci* 1994; 91: 11889-93.
11. Winberg J, Möllby R, Bergström J, Karlsson KA, Leonardsson I, Milh M, Teneberg S, Haslam D, Marklund BI, Normark S. *J Exp Med* 1995; 182: 1695-702.
12. Bock K, Breimer M, Brignole A, Hansson G, Karlsson KA, Larsson G, Leffler H, Samuelsson B, Strömberg N, Svanborg-Edén C, Thurin J. *J Biol Chem* 1985; 260: 8545-51.
13. Breimer M, Hansson G, Leffler H. *J Biochem* 1985; 98: 1169-80.
14. Lomberg H, Svanborg-Edén C. *FEMS Microbiol Immunol* 1989; 47: 363-70.
15. Lindberg F, Lund B, Johansson L, Normark S. *Nature* 1987; 328: 84-7.
16. Lund B, Marklund BI, Strömberg N, Lindberg F, Karlsson K, Normark S. *Mol Microbiol* 1988; 2: 255-63.
17. Strömberg N, Marklund BI, Lund B, Ilver D, Hamers A, Gaastra W, Karlsson KA, Normark S. *EMBO J* 1990; 9: 2001-10.
18. Lindstedt R, Falk P, Hull R, Hull S, Leffler H, Svanborg-Edén C, Larson G. *Infect Immun* 1989; 57: 3389-94.
19. Johanson I, Lindstedt R, Svanborg C. *Infect Immun* 1992; 60: 3416-22.
20. Plos K, Carter T, Hull S, Hull R, Svanborg-Edén C. *J Infect Dis* 1990; 161: 518-24.
21. Johanson IM, Plos K, Marklund BI, Svanborg C. *Microbiol Path* 1993; 15: 121-9.

22. Hedges S, Anderson P, Lidin-Janson G, De Man P, Svanborg C. *Infect Immun* 1991; 59: 421-7.
23. Agace W, Hedges S, Ceska M, Svanborg C. *J Clin Invest* 1993; 92: 780-5.
24. Svensson M, Lindstedt R, Radin N, Svanborg C. *Infect Immun* 1994; 62: 4404-10.
25. Hedges S, Svensson M, Svanborg C. *Infect Immun* 1992; 60: 1295-301.
26. Okazaki T, Bell RM, Hannun YA. *J Biol Chem* 1989; 264: 19076-80.
27. Kim MY, Linardic C, Obeid LM, Hannun YA. *J Biol Chem* 1991; 266: 484-9.
28. Dressler KA, Mathias S, Kolesnick RN. *Science* 1992; 255: 1715-8.
29. Hedlund M, Sevensson M, Nilsson A, Duan RD, Svanborg C. *J Exp Med* 1996; 247: 1037-44.
30. Mathias S, Dressler KA, Kolesnick RN. *Proc Natl Acad Sci USA* 1991; 88: 10009-13.
31. Raines MA, Kolesnick RN, Golde DW. *J Biol Chem* 1993; 268: 14572-5.
32. Schütze S, Potthoff K, Machleidt T, Berkovic C, Wiegman K, Krönke M. *Cell* 1992; 71: 765-76.
33. Mathias S, Younes A, Kan C, Orlow I, Joseph C, Kolesnick R. *Science* (Wash. DC) 1993; 259: 519-22.
34. Cifone M, De Maria R, Roncaioli P, Rippo M, Azuma M, Lanier L, Santini A, Testi R. *J Exp Med* 1993; 177: 1547-52.
35. Somerville JE Jr, Cassiano L, Bainbridge B, Cunningham MD, Darveau R. *J Clin Invest* 1996; 997: 359-65.
36. Joseph C, Wright S, Bornmann W, Randolph J, Kumar E, Bittman R, Liu J, Kolesnick R. *J Biol Chem* 1994; 269: 17606-10.
37. Linder H, Engberg I, Mattsby-Baltzer I, Svanborg-Edén C. *FEMS Microbiol Lett* 1988; 49: 219-22.
38. Brauner A, Svenson SB, Wretlind B, Julander I, Källenius G, Leissner M. *Eur J Clin Microbiol* 1985; 4: 566-9.
39. Johnson JR, Roberts PL, Stamm WE. *J Infect Dis* 1987; 156: 225-9.
40. Otto G, Sandberg T, Marklund BI, Ulleryd P, Svanborg C. *Clin Infect Dis* 1993; 17: 448-56.
41. Giard DJ, Aaronson SA, Todaro GJ, Arnstein P, Kersey JH, Dosik H, Parks WP. *J Natl Cancer Inst* 1973; 51: 1417-23.
42. Lund B, Lindberg F, Båge M, Nordmark S. *J Bacteriol* 1985; 162: 1293-301.
43. Lund B, Lindberg F, Marklund BI, Nordmark S. *Mol Microbiol* 1987; 84: 5898-902.
44. Otto G, Sandberg T, Marklund BI, Ulleryd P, Svanborg C. *Clin Infect Dis* 1993; 17: 448-56.
45. Hull R, Gill RE, Hsu P, Minshew BH, Falkow S. *Infect Immun* 1981; 33: 933-8.
46. Aronso M, Medalia O, Amichay D, Nativ O. *Infect Immun* 1988; 56: 1615-7.
47. Eckmann L, Kagnoff MF, Fierer J. *Infect Immun* 1993; 61: 4569-74.
48. Metcalf ES, O'Neill BL, Hone DM, Kaiserlian D, Weinstein DL. *Clin Immunol Immunopath* 1995; 76 (1) Part 2: S101; 593.
49. Agace W, Patarroyo M, Svensson M, Carlemalm E, Svanborg C. *Infect Immun* 1995; 63 (10): 4045-62.
50. Godaly G, Offord R, Proudfoot A, Svanborg C, Agace W. *Infect Immun* 1997; 65: 3451-6.
51. Godaly G, Frendéus B, Agace WW, Proudfoot A, Svensson M, Klemm P, Svanborg C. *Mol Microb* 1998; submitted.
52. Lindberg U. *Acta Paediatr Scand* 1975; 64: 718-24.
53. Hansson S, Caugant D, Jodal U, Svanborg-Edén C. *Br Med J* 1989; 298: 853-5.
54. Hagberg L, Bruce A, Reid G, Svanborg-Edén C, Lincoln K, Lidin-Janson G. In: Kass E, Svanborg-Edén C, eds. Host-Parasite Interactions. In: *Urinary Tract Infections*. Chicago: Chicago Press, 1986: 194-297.
55. Anderson P, Engberg I, Lidin-Janson G, Lincoln K, Hull R, Hull S, Svanborg-Edén C. *Infect Immun* 1991; 59: 2915-21.
56. Otto G, Braconier JH, Andreasson A, Svanborg C. *J Infect Dis* 1998; in press.

57. Rogers H, Unanue E. *Infect Immun* 1993; 61: 5090.
58. Conlan J, North R. *J Exp Med* 1994; 179: 259.
59. Conlan JW, North RJ. *J Leukoc Biol* 1992; 52: 130.
60. Conlan JW, North RJ. *Infect Immun* 1994; 62: 2779.
61. O'Brien A, Weinstein DL, Soliman MY, Rosensteich DL. *J Immunol* 1985; 134: 2820.
62. Svanborg-Edén C, Shahin R, Briles D. *J Immunol* 1988; 140: 3180.
63. Shahin RD, Engberg I, Hagberg L, Svanborg-Edén C. *J Immunol* 1987; 138 (10): 3475-80.

Invasive bacteria in the gastrointestinal tract

Recent advances in the pathogenesis of gastrointestinal bacterial infections.
P. Rampal, P. Boquet, eds. John Libbey Eurotext, Paris © 1998, pp. 83-95.

Mechanisms of *Shigella* invasion

Guy Tran Van Nhieu, Philippe Sansonetti

Unité de Pathogénie Microbienne Moléculaire, INSERM U 389, Institut Pasteur, 28, rue du Docteur-Roux, 75724 Paris Cedex 15, France

Shigella spp. are foodborn pathogens responsible for acute intestinal infections in humans, with clinical manifestations ranging from mild watery diarrhoea to the dysenteric syndrome, a severe diarrhoea with the emission of blood and mucus in the stools. This severe form of shigellosis accounts for a significant percentage of death related to diarrhoeal diseases, specially among young infants in developing countries. Two species are mainly responsible for severe dysentery: *Shigella dysenteriae* and *Shigella flexneri. S. dysenteriae* serotype 1, the most virulent strain, is associated with epidemics, whereas *S. flexneri* is the major species associated with the endemic form of the disease. *S. boydii* and *S. sonnei* are responsible for milder forms of shigellosis, most often represented by self-limiting watery diarrhoea. Watery diarrhoea linked to shigellosis is usually associated with fluid secretion at the level of the proximal jejunum without major lesions of the intestinal mucosa. Dysentery, on the other hand, corresponds to an intense inflammatory reaction at the level of the colon and rectum, linked to *Shigella* invasion of the colonic epithelium, leading to destruction of the mucosa.

Shigella infections are specific for humans and with the exception of naturally infectable hosts such as monkeys, most common laboratory animals are resistant to *Shigella* infection. As opposed to other enteropathogens, the infectious dose required for the establishment of shigellosis is extremely low in humans and ingestion of as little as a few hundreds bacteria is sufficient to initiate the disease. Animal models for shigellosis, on the other hand, usually imply important input of bacteria to trigger host inflammatory responses, and attempts to reconstitute the disease in animal models may not faithfully reproduce natural symptoms. There are currently three models to test for virulence of *Shigella* strains in animals. These consist of the mouse pulmonary infection, the guinea pig corneal epithelium (Sereny test), and the rabbit small intestine. This latter, which may represent the most physiologically relevant model for shigellosis, has been used to study various parameters linked to the inflammation of the intestinal mucosa induced by *Shigella* (*i.e.:* height/width ratio of the villosity, fluid secretion, cytokine production, polymorphonuclear leucocyte counts...). These models, in combination with *in vitro* cultured cell systems, have allowed the characterization of several *Shigella* determinants that are crucial for its virulence.

Shigella invasion of cultured cells

Shigella spp. are gram-negative bacteria which are genetically highly homologous to *E. coli.* Virulence, however, is associated with the presence of a large plasmid which determines the invasion abilities of these pathogens. This makes of *Shigella* an amenable model to genetically study virulence determinants. Among these determinants, the ability of *Shigella* to invade normally non-phagocytic cells, as well as to spread from cell-to-cell within an epithelium stand out as particularly important features for the virulence of these bacteria. These *Shigella* properties have been studied using cultured cells and microscopic observations in such systems have allowed to distinguish subsequent steps in the cell invasion process. *Shigella* induces its internalization by triggering localized deformations of the cell membrane in a process resembling macropinocytosis. After internalization by the cell, *Shigella* lyse the phagocytic vacuole and multiply freely within the cell cytosol. During this replication phase, *Shigella* polymerizes cellular actin to move intracellularly. This actin-based motility allows the formation of bacteria-containing protrusions originating from *Shigella* infected cells, which can invade neighbouring cells. The bacteria contained in the protrusions then lyse the double-membrane of the donor and recipient cell and the cycle of infection can resume. By repeating this infectious cycle, *Shigella* can potentially spread within an epithelium without extracellular steps. Such intercellular spreading properties have been also developed by other pathogens, such as *Listeria*, and may allow colonization of an epithelium by microorganisms that are protected from host humoral responses by their intracellular location.

Entry *via* M cells and macrophage-induced apopotosis: a model for tissular invasion by *Shigella*

Using polarized cultured cells, such as Caco-2 or T84 cells, it became clear that *Shigella* could not efficiently invade epithelial cells *via* the apical side. To get successful *Shigella* invasion of these polarized cells required to pretreat the cells with a divalent cation chelator to open intercellular junctions, or to challenge the cells with *Shigella via* their basal side using cells grown on transwell filters [1]. These results raised a paradox as *in vivo*, the initial steps of infection require interactions of microorganisms present in the lumen of the intestinal tract with the surface of intestinal mucosa. When a *Shigella* mutant strain that was deficient for cell-to-cell spread was used to orally infect macaque monkeys, it was found that during the early phases of infection, *Shigella* does not invade the colonic mucosa *via* the enterocytes' brush border, but at the level of M cells [2]. M cells are specialized cells of the intestinal epithelium, which overlay solitary lymph nodes or lymphoid follicles (Peyer's patches); their presumed role is to sample antigens from the intestinal lumen to present them to the immune system. Several enteropathogens appear to target M cells to breach the intestinal epithelial layer; although the reasons for this preferential tropism are not clear, several particularities of M cells may explain this. First, M cells are considered to be somewhat phagocytic. This property by itself does not exclude the necessity for enteroinvasive pathogens to express entry determinants, but it may contribute to the invasion process. As opposed to enterocytes, M cells have a poorly organized brush border and do not secrete mucus; the absence of such features which could represent a mechanical hindrance for enteropathogens, may explain the fact that they are preferentially targeted. Finally, M cells do not appear to show the same levels of polarization as enterocytes; for example, surface markers, such as the sucrase isomaltase, show a different distribution on M cells than on neighbouring enterocytes. Although this remain to be firmly established, it is likely that M cells express surface receptors on their apical side that are different than those present on the surface of enterocytes. Perhaps, some of these receptors which are distributed basolaterally on enterocytes, are accessible on the apical surface of M cells and act as receptors for pathogens.

Pathogens that invade the epithelium *via* M cells need to develop ways to survive cells of the immune system. Resident macrophages, which are often found in pockets underlying M cells, probably constitute the first line of defense of the host. As this seems to hold true for many other enteropathogens, *Shigella* has the ability to kill the macrophage by inducing an apoptotic process [3]. In the case of *Shigella*, however, bacterial-induced apoptosis may not be a mean for the invading organism to depress the inflammatory response, but rather can be used to trigger a specific inflammation that favors the colonization of the colonic mucosa by *Shigella*. Macrophage infected by *Shigella* undergo apoptosis after activation of the ICE-cysteine protease, which converts pro-IL 1 to mature IL-1 proteolytic cleavage. The release of the pro-inflammatory IL-1 cytokine by macrophage undergoing apoptosis results in an influx of circulating monocytes and polynuclear from blood vessels to the site of infection, thus destabilizing the epithelium *(figure 1)*. The epithelium destabilization and opening of intercellular junctions then favors superinfection by bacteria present in the lumen of the intestine *(figure 1)*. The intense inflammatory response is primarily responsible for the destruction of the colonic mucosa induced by *Shigella*. Studies using ileal loops of rabbits that were perfused with an IL-1 receptor antagonist indicated that when IL-1 dependent responses were impaired, the intestinal mucosa did not show significant alterations upon challenge with *Shigella*. It therefore appears that the establishment of the disease requires the capacity by the infected tissues to induce inflammatory responses, and that *Shigella* may further use this inflammatory reaction to colonize the mucosal epithelium.

Shigella invasive determinants: an overview

The use of cultured cell systems in combination with genetic analysis of *Shigella* mutants have led to the identification of several genes required for invasion and dissemination in epithelial cells. Although probably not exhaustive, the characterization of the these genes and of phenotypes associated with their inactivation has unveiled some specific features about interactions between *Shigella* and host cells.

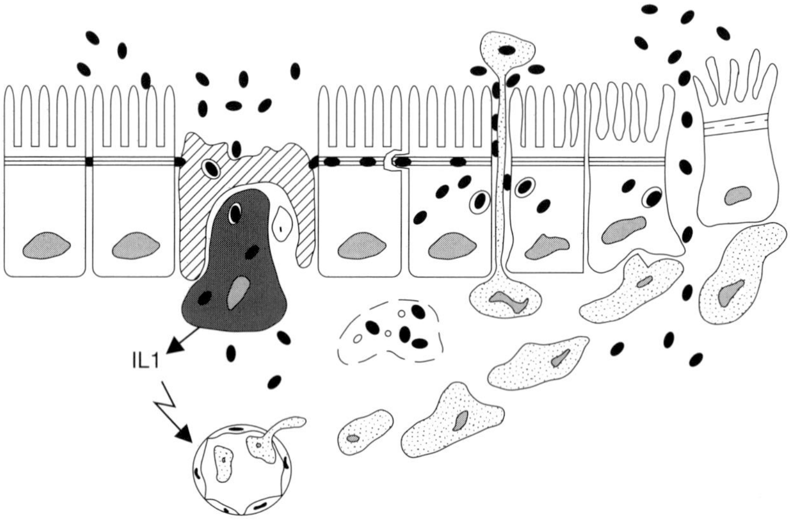

Figure 1. *Shigella* invasion of the colonic epithelium. *Shigella* first invades the epithelium at the level of M cells (hatched lines), which are cells specialized in the sampling of antigens from the lumen of the intestine. After internalization by M cells, *Shigella* kills the macrophage (black) in apoptotic process that results in synthesis of IL-1, a pro-inflammatory cytokine with chemotactic activity towards monocytes and polymorphonuclear cells (dotted lines). The influx of monocytes from efferent blood vessels contributes to the destabilization of the epithelium, and favors further infection of enterocytes (white) by bacteria present in the lumen of the intestine. A combination of *Shigella* invasive determinants and the host inflammatory response leads to destruction of the colonic mucosa. (Figure from Zineb Ben Jelloum, 1997, doctoral dissertation.)

The Ipa proteins as determinants of cell entry

The ability of *Shigella* to enter epithelial cells is determined by a 30 kb region of the virulence plasmid which encompasses up to 30 different genes [4]. This region can be subdivided in two transcription units (operons) that are divergently transcribed, the *mxi-spa* operon and the *ipa* operon. The mxi-spa operon encodes a type III secretion apparatus for which homologs have been identified in many gram-negative bacteria that are pathogenic for mammalians hosts or plants. An increasing body of evidence suggests that this specialized secretion apparatus allows translocation of bacterial effectors from the extracellular bacteria to the cell cytosol upon cell contact [5]. Probably the best characterized system is the *Yersinia* Ysc type III secretion apparatus (see Cornelis *et al.*, this issue). Upon contact with host cells, the *Yersinia* Yop proteins are secreted *via* the Ysc secretory apparatus. One of them, the YopB protein, may form a pore across the host cell membrane through which other Yop proteins, such as YopH and YopE, translocate from the extracellular bacteria to the macrophage cytosol to inihibit phagocytosis [5]. In the case of *Shigella*, the Ipa proteins are secreted *via* the Mxi-Spa secretion apparatus upon cell contact. As opposed to the Yop proteins for which expression induced upon cell contact, the *Shigella* Ipa proteins are expressed during bacterial growth *in vitro*, and are stored unfolded in the bacterial cytoplasm [6]: upon cell contact, the Ipa proteins are secreted within seconds and important amounts can readily be detected in the culture medium. It is believed that this massive and rapid secretion conditions the entry process. The Ipa operon encodes four Ipa proteins (IpaA-D), and non-polar mutagenesis of the corresponding genes indicate that they are all involved in cell entry. IpaB, C and D are critical for the entry process [7], whereas IpaA appears to optimize the entry efficiency [8]. IpaB and IpaD also appear to play a role in regulating secretion, as the corresponding mutants show a constitutive secretion of the Mxi-Spa secretory apparatus [9]. More direct evidences implicate IpaB and IpaC, which associate extracellularly, in the entry process. Inert particles, such as latex beads, coated with the IpaB, C complex are readily internalized by cultured cells, suggesting that these invasins may be the actual effectors of *Shigella* entry [10]. The putative mode of action of these different *Shigella* effectors of entry will be discussed further.

Determinants of intercellular spread

To spread from cell-to-cell, *Shigella* must lyse the phagocytic vacuole, replicate intracellularly and move within the cell cytosol. Many genes are required for intracellular replication of *Shigella*. Some of them, such as auxotrophic markers or genes encoding siderophores, appear to affect the general bacterial physiology [2]. Also, some genes may be involved in DNA replication and bacterial septation when multiplying intracellularly, but not when grown extracellularly [11]. Such genes are probably representative of the bacterial adaptation to the intracellular environment, involving complex interconnections between the host and the bacterial metabolism. Their denomination as virulence determinants is a matter of debate, because rather than performing specific functions required for producing the disease, they may favor bacterial growth under conditions which may not be strictly specific for the host.

A lot of attention has been focused on *Shigella* determinants that are involved in more specific steps of the *Shigella* intracellular cycle. Interestingly, the IpaB and IpaC invasins which are required for the cell entry process, have also been implicated in the lysis of the phagocytic vacuole. It is not clear if this reflets an activity linked to these proteins that is distinct from the one required for cell entry. Part of the limitation of mutant analysis, is the ability to distinguish between specific effects linked to a particular effector, or broader effects linked to a defect in a bacterial component. For example, IpaB is critical for *Shigella* entry into cells, but IpaB also regulates the secretion of other effectors. Also, efforts aiming at delineating subdomains of Ipa proteins involved in secretion, entry, or vacuole lysis, have been so far unconclusive due to intrinsec difficulty of manipulating these genes without altering expression. There are conflicting evidences about a role for IpaB in the lysis of the vacuole, some of which may come from the cell line studied. In epithelial cells, however, IpaB may not be directly linked to vacuole lysis. For example, *Salmonella*, another enteropathogen responsible for diarrheal diseases, enters epithelial cells using a strategy that is similar to *Shigella*, with the Salmonella Sip proteins sharing significiant homologies with the *Shigella* Ipa proteins. As opposed to *Shigella*, however, *Salmonella* does not lyse the vacuole after internalization by the cell and remains confined within large vacuole where it multiplies. Complementation of a *Shigella ipaB* mutant with a copy of SipB, its *Salmonella* homologous counterpart, result in a *Shigella* strain that lyses the phagocytic vacuole [12]. These results suggest that rather than being actively involved in the lysis, IpaB allows proper targeting of IpaC and perhaps other bacterial effectors with haemolytic activity towards the vacuolar membrane.

Once escaped from the vacuole, *Shigella* needs to lyse a cell membrane with supposedly an inverted polarity to infect neighbouring cells. The *vacJ* and *icsB* genes have been implicated in the lysis of the protrusion membrane [13, 14], and their products may have such an activity although this remains speculative at this point.

Many efforts have been made to analyze the mechanisms of *Shigella* actin-based motility. Beside its obvious interests in terms of pathology, the actin-based motility of intracellular organisms such as *Listeria* (see Cossart *et al.*, this issue) or *Shigella*, provide interesting models to study the dynamics of the cell cytoskeleton. Central to *Shigella* intracellular motility is the expression of IcsA (also called VirG) at the surface of the bacterium. The IcsA protein, which has the particularity to be localized at one pole of the bacterial body, is directly responsible for the polymerization of actin that drives *Shigella* motility *(figure 2)* [15]. *Shigella* mutants that are defective for IcsA expression are still able to invade epithelial cells and to lyse the phagocytic vacuole, but are unable to move intracellularly and to spread from cell-to-cell. As a consequence, *icsA* mutants are unable to induce keratocunjunctivitis in guinea pigs and are avirulent in the rabbit ileal loop model. Also, polarization of IcsA at one pole of the bacterium appears to be critical for actin-based motility. For example, LPS mutants of *Shigella* or a mutant of *Shigella* defective for SopA, a protease cleaving IcsA, express IcsA on the bacterial surface but are not able to polarize it at one pole of the bacterial body [16]. Such mutants are also affected for cell-to-cell spread.

IcsA is encoded by the *Shigella* large virulence plasmid and under its mature form, consists of a 120 kDa protein with two-third of its N-terminal part (α-domain) being exposed on the surface, the C-terminal part (β-domain) being necessary for the translocation and anchoring of the α-domain on the bacterial surface. The α-domain bears the actin polymerization activity and can be further subdivided into two regions: i) a region containing glycine-rich repeats, which is required for the nucleation of actin; ii) a region which allows the organization of actin filaments into an actin comet tail-like structure. Interestingly, the IcsA α-domain has been shown to bind vinculin, a focal adhesion component which is presumed to anchor the cytoskeleton to the plasma membrane [17]. Both activities are required for motility, but little is known about their precise role in this process. It has been proposed that binding of IcsA to the head domain of vinculin favors actin polymerization by allowing recruitment of VASP [18], another focal adhesion component that binds profilin, aG-actin binding protein with potential actin polymerization activity. In fact, there is little consensus on the mechanism of IcsA induced actin polymerization, as actin polymerization can occur in the absence of vinculin. Reasons for this may be the existence of redundant cellular pathways that lead to actin polymerization.

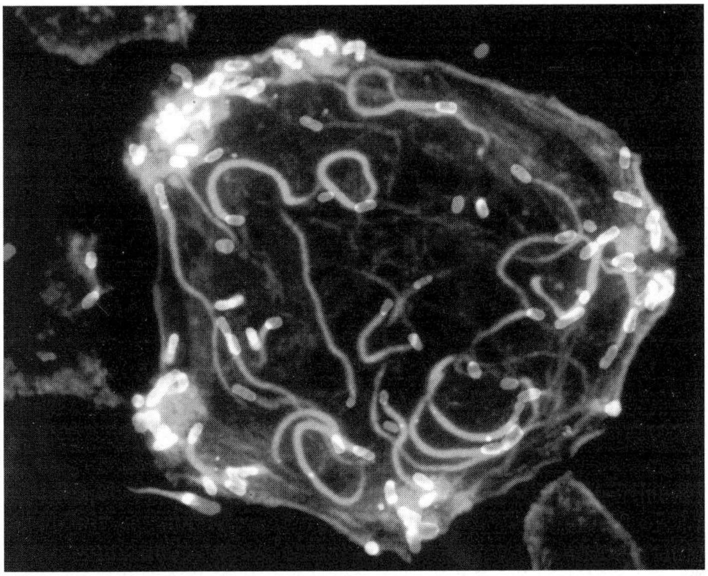

Figure 2. Intracellular multiplication and actin-based motility of *Shigella.* Cultured HeLa cells were challenged with *Shigella,* and gentamicin was added to the medium to prevent multiplication of extracellular bacteria. After incubation for a few hours to allow intracellular multiplication of *Shigella,* samples were fixed and process for immunofluorescence staining using anti-LPS antibody to label bacteria, or fluorescein-labeled phallacidin to stain F-actin. Polymerization of actin in a "comet-tail" structure is visible at one pole of the bacterium, and provides the driving force for *Shigella's* intracellular motility. (Courtesy from Coumaran Egile, Institut Pasteur, Paris, France.)

Shigella invasion of epithelial cells: a cellular view

Cytoskeletal rearrangements also play a major role during *Shigella* entry. Staining of F-actin in cell samples challenged with *Shigella* indicate an area of intense actin polymerization in the vicinity of the bacteria in the process of inducing its internalization. Moreover, cell treatment with inhibitor of F-actin such as the cytochalasins, results in complete inhibition of *Shigella* uptake by epithelial cells, indicating that actin polymerization is critical for the entry process. It is believed that actin polymerization induced by *Shigella* at the site of entry drives the formation of cellular extensions that raise above the cell surface and fuse to engulf the bacterial body in a large vacuole. Indeed, electron microscopy of entry structures labeled with myosin S1 headpiece indicates that the *Shigella*-induced extensions contain actin filaments in parallel orientation, with their barbed end mostly facing the membrane [19]. As addition of actin monomers occurs at the free barbed end of filaments, these observations suggest that actin polymerization by itself is responsible for the elongation of cell extensions.

To investigate the molecular mechanisms involved in *Shigella*-induced actin rearrangements, the effects on inhibition of Rho proteins have been analyzed. The Rho subfamily are small GTPases which regulate specific cytoskeletal rearrangements [20]. They consist of three related members, Cdc42, Rac and Rho itself. Cdc42 and Rac activation lead to actin polymerization in structures at the cell periphery. Cdc42 determines the formation of microspikes and filopodia, whereas Rac appears to be mostly responsible for lamellipodia formation. Rho on the other hand, is mostly implied in the formation of focal adhesions and stress fibers, which do not appear to require actin polymerization. These GTPases can be inhibited by expression of a dominant negative form, bearing a mutation in an asparagine residue in position 17 for Cdc42 and Rac, or in position 19 for Rho. Using such constructs, it was shown that Cdc42 and Rac was required for *Shigella* entry (Mounier *et al.*, submitted). Transient expression of a dominant negative form of Rac or Cdc42 in HeLa cells leads to an inhibition of *Shigella* entry by approximately 70%. The reduction in entry in these cells corresponds to the unability of *Shigella* to induce actin polymerization upon interaction with the cell membrane. In instances where polymerization occurred, the levels of polymerization were clearly affected. These results indicate that the *Shigella* Ipa proteins activate Cdc42 and Rac upon entry and that both are required for the entry process. Perhaps more surprising was the finding that Rho was also critical for the entry process, as Rho is not classically involved in ruffling-like responses. Rho can be specifically inhibited by the C3 exoenzyme from *Clostridium botulinum* by ADP-ribosylation on asparagine 41. Cell treatment with C3 resulted in 90% inhibition of *Shigella* entry. *Shigella*-induced actin polymerization in these cells was also inhibited, although some nucleation of actin filaments was still detectable at the very close vicinity of the bacterium interacting with the cell membrane [21]. It therefore appears that all three Rho proteins are required for *Shigella* entry process, although detailed analysis may indicate various levels of participation of the different small GTPases. Activation of these proteins probably directs actin rearrangements as well as the recruitment of cytoskeletal proteins required for *Shigella* entry structures.

Among the cytoskeletal proteins recruited at the site of *Shigella* entry, actin bundling proteins, such as α-actinin or plastin, may constitute scaffolding proteins that stabilize the cellular extensions as they raise above the bacterial body [19]. Recently, ezrin, a member of the ERM family of proteins that act as membrane-cytoskeletal linkers, has been localized at the tip of the cellular extensions (Skoudy *et al.*, submitted). Ezrin is required for *Shigella* entry, and may be directly involved in the induction of membrane deformations induced by *Shigella* at the entry site. Also, focal adhesion components, such as vinculin or talin, are recruited at the site of *Shigella* entry. In this latter case, however, these components appear to show a distinct sublocalization in the entry site, as they show a preferential recruitment at the close vicinity of the membrane juxtaposing the bacterium in the process of internalization. This specific localization was shown to be dependent on IpaA, a *Shigella* invasin that directly binds vinculin [8]. This interaction between IpaA and vinculin is not critical for the entry process and for *Shigella* induced actin polymerization, but increases the entry efficiency by up to two orders of magnitude. It is speculated that translocation of IpaA from *Shigella* in the cell cytosol during the entry process permits the transformation of a primary actin polymerization response. IpaB and IpaC would be responsible for the initial induction of actin polymerization at the level of the entry site, but in this case, the cellular extensions produced resembles microspikes and do not appear to be productive for *Shigella* internalization *(figure 3)*. IpaA interaction with vinculin would modulate this primary response, and convert this microspike-like extensions into membrane leaflets by conditionning the recruitment of actin-bundling proteins. The formation of the vinculin/talin rich region at the intimate contact with the bacterium is also dependent on IpaA: this particular region has been referred to as a pseudo-focal adhesion which may favor stabilization of *Shigella* within the foci of entry, and which could also play a role in the pulling of the bacterium within the cell body *(figure 3)*.

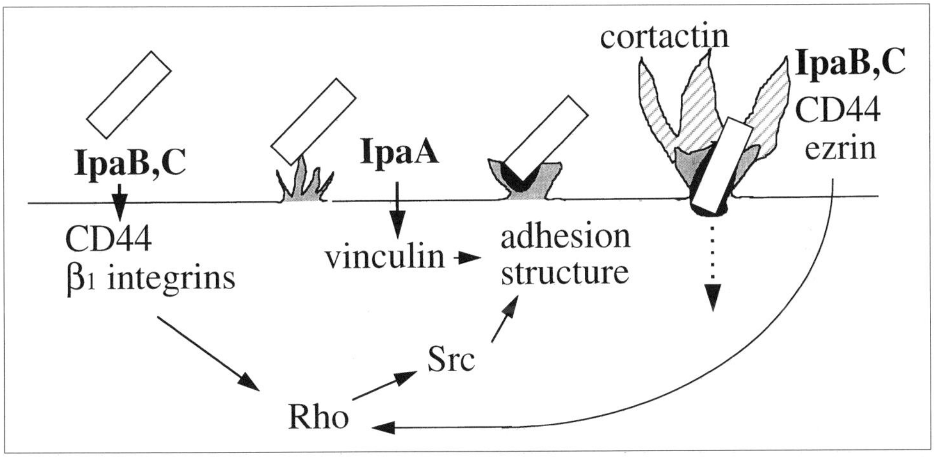

Figure 3. Different steps during *Shigella* invasion of epithelial cells. The *Shigella* Ipa proteins determine the entry process. IpaB and IpaC are responsible for the primary cell response that leads to actin polymerization. Binding of IpaB to CD44 and β1 integrins receptors appears to be important for the process, and may allow access to the cytosol of IpaA and IpaC. Activation of Rho proteins and of the Src tyrosine kinase is required for the formation of microspike-like extensions (shaded in grey) at the site of bacterial interaction with the cell membrane. Interaction between IpaA and vinculin further regulates cytoskeletal reorganization by allowing the formation of an F-actin network, rich in vinculin, and talin, at the immediate vicinity of the membrane contacting the bacterium (solid area), as well as the recruitment of the actin bundling protein α-actinin in the extensions. During the late stages of foci formation, ezrin and cortactin are preferentially recruited in the tip of the extensions, where little polymerization of actin is detected (hatched area). The Ipa proteins act in concert to induce membrane deformations that are productive for the efficient internalization of *Shigella*.

Substrates for the tyrosine kinase Src, as well as Src itself, are also recruited at the site of *Shigella* entry. This is of particular interest as Src has also been implicated in the formation of focal adhesions further suggesting that *Shigella* entry and focal adhesion formation share similar processes. In the case of focal adhesion formation, however, the kinase activity of Src does not appear to be required, as Src may mostly allow recruitment of its substrates such as FAK, or paxillin, *via* its SH2 and SH3 domain. In contrast, several lines of evidence indicate that Src activation and catalytic activity is required for *Shigella* entry. First, cortactin, an actin binding protein that is a substrate for Src, is specifically tyrosylphosphorylated upon *Shigella* entry [22]. Overexpression of an active form of Src in cells leads to hyperphosphorylation of cortactin by *Shigella* entry. Finally, expression of a dominant negative form of Src that bears a mutation in its catalytic domain, results in an inhibition of cortactin phosphorylation as well as inhibition of the cytoskeletal rearrangements induced by *Shigella* (Duménil *et al.* submitted). The precise role of Src activation during *Shigella* entry is yet to be characterized: Src could activate cytoskeletal components that are required for actin rearrangements, but it may also participate in the coordination of subsequent steps occurring during foci formation.

Shigella Ipa proteins and cell invasion

As mentionned previous ly, the *Shigella* IpaB and IpaC proteins are directly responsible for the entry process. These proteins are secreted upon cell contact and an important fraction can be recovered in the cell medium under the form of an IpaB-IpaC complex. Affinity chromatography approaches using purified Ipa proteins or recombinant Ipa proteins indicate that the IpaB-C complex can associate with β1 integrins, which are receptors for the extracellular matrix. These findings were particularly interesting because in some instances, β1 integrins can associate with the actin cytoskeleton *via* the cytoplasmic tail of the integrin β1 subunit. Also, bacterial binding to these receptors had been shown to result in bacterial internalization. For example, binding of the *Yersinia* surface protein invasion to β1 integrins leads to bacterial internationalization in a zipper-like process [23]. In this particular case, however, entry correlates with a tight bacterial attachment to the cell surface. Internalization occurs with the formation of cell pseudopods in tight apposition with the bacterial body and results in engulfment of the bacterium in a tight vacuole. It is believed that incremental interactions between the Invasin protein and β1 integrins drive the extension of the cell pseudopods, in a process highly dependent on receptor-ligand affinity. This is in contrast to what is observed during *Shigella*, as tight attachment does not seem to be a prerequisite for cell entry. Furthermore, membrane deformations (ruffles) induced by *Shigella* occur in a cell area wich extend beyond the site of bacteria interaction with the cell membrane. It is therefore likely that mere binding of the IpaB-C complex to β1 entegrins is not sufficient to trigger te entry process. More recently, using a similar affinity chromatography procedure, it was found that IpaB could directly bind CD44, the hyaluronan receptor (Skoudy *et al.*, submitted). Interestingly, CD44 can associate *via* its cytoplasmic tail with proteins from the ERM family, including ezrin. This led to speculation that IpaB binding to CD44 determines ezrin recruitment at *Shigella* entry structures *(figure 3)*. As ezrin can also associate with actin filaments upon activation, the IpaB-CD44 interaction in combination with IpaB-C interaction with β1 integrins may induce the cytoskeletal rearrangements observed at the site of entry. A few observations, however, are inconsistent with the notion that binding of IpaB to surface receptors is sufficient to promote *Shigella*-induced membrane rearrangements during entry. First, addition of the purified IpaB protein to cultured cells does not have any significant effect on the cell cytoskeleton. Also, inhibitors, such as kinase inhibitors, that shut off transduction pathways triggered upon receptor engagement to physiological stimuli, have little effect on *Shigella* entry. Finally, *Shigella* mutants that are deficient for IpaB or IpaC are totally deficient for entry, whereas cell lines that do not express β1 integrins or CD44 are still sensitive to *Shigella* invasion (Skoudy, unpublished). Binding of IpaB-C to surface receptors may represent only a discrete view of the entry process, and it is possible that this binding is required for the activity of other Ipa proteins. By analogy with type III secretion apparatus found in other enteropathogens, it is possible that Ipa proteins are translocated into the cell cytosol to induce actin rearrangements. Some levels of homology between the *Yersinia* and *Shigella* type III secretion systems argue for this, as the *Shigella* IpaB protein can be secreted by *Yersinia in vitro* [24]. IpaB may permit translocation of other Ipa proteins in the cell cytosol. In this case, however, these Ipa proteins may stimulate actin rearrangements that lead to *Shigella* uptake. There are some evidences that this is the case for IpaA, as IpaA binding to vinculin is detected early during the entry process, and IpaA can be immunolocalized in membrane deformations induced by extracellular *Shigella*. Perhaps access to the cell cytosol for bacterial effectors, such as IpaC is also required to induce initial cytoskeletal rearrangements.

Conclusions

The analysis of the mode of action of *Shigella* determinants that allow colonization of the epithelium underlines that this bacterial pathogen can divert host cell responses at several levels. At a tissular level, divertion of the host inflammatory responses *via* local control of cytokine production may also serve to the establishment of the disease. At a cellular level, determinants of invasion and cell-to-cell spread appear to specifically target regulators of the actin cytoskeleton, or cytoskeletal proteins themselves. Analysis of the molecular mechanisms involved in the divertion of host cell functions during the entry and the cell-to-cell spreading process of *Shigella* is likely to bring important clues on the regulation of actin dynamics that condition cell fundamental processes, such as cellular adhesion and motility.

References

1. Mounier J, Vasselon T, Hellio R, Lesourd M, Sansonetti PJ. *Shigella flexneri* enters human colonic Caco-2 epithelial cells through the basolateral pole. *Infect Immun* 1992; 60: 237-8.
2. Sansonetti PJ. Molecular mechanisms of cell and tissue invasion by *Shigella flexneri. Infect Agents Dis* 1993; 2: 201-6.

3. Zychlinsky A, Sansonetti PJ. Apoptose, interleukine-1 et shigellose. *Med Sci* 1995; 11: 128-9.
4. Parsot C. *Shigella flexneri*: genetics of entry and intercellular dissemination in epithelial cells. *Bacterial pathogenesis of plants and animals, molecular and cellular mechanisms*. In : Dangl JL, Springer Verlag, 1994: 217-41.
5. Cornelis G, Wolf-Watz H. The *Yersinia* Yop virulon: a bacterial system for subverting eukaryotic cells. *Mol Microbiol* 1997; 23: 861-7.
6. Ménard R, Sansonetti PJ, Parsot C, Vasselon T. Extracellular association and cytoplasmic partitioning of the IpaB and IpaC invasins of *Shigella flexneri. Cell* 1994a; 79: 515-25.
7. Ménard R, Sansonetti PJ, Parsot C. Non polar mutagenesis of the *ipa* gene defines IpaB, IpaC and IpaD as effectors of *Shigella flexneri* entry into epithelial cells. *J Bacteriol* 1993; 175: 5899-906.
8. Tran Van Nhieu G, Ben Ze'ev A, Sansonetti PJ. Modulation of bacterial entry into epithelial cells by interaction between vinculin and the *Shigella* IpaA invasin. *EMBO J* 1997 (in press).
9. Parsot C, Ménard R, Gounon P, Sansonetti PJ. Enhanced secretion through the *Shigella flexneri* Mxi-Spa translocon leads to assembly of extracellular proteins into macromolecular structures. *Mol Microbiol* 1995; 16: 291-300.
10. Ménard R, Prévost MC, Gounon P, Sansonetti P, Dehio C. The secreted Ipa complex of *Shigella flexneri* promotes entry into mammalian cells. *Proc Natl Acad Sci USA* 1996; 93: 1254-8.
11. Mac Siomoin RA, Nakata N, Murai T, Yoshikawa M, Tsuji H, Sasakawa C. Identification and characterization of ispA, a *Shigella flexneri* chromosomal gene essential for normal *in vivo* cell division and intracellular spreading. *Mol Microbiol* 1996; 16: 599-609.
12. Hermant D, Ménard N, Arricau N, Parsot C, Popoff MY. Functional conservation of the *Salmonella* and *Shigella* effectors of entry into epithelial cells. *Mol Microbiol* 1995: 781-9.
13. Allaoui A, Mounier J, Prévost MC, Sansonetti PJ, Parsot C. *icsB*: a *S. flexneri* virulence gene necessary for the lysis of protrusions during intercellular spread. *Mol Microbiol* 1992c; 6: 1605-16.
14. Suzuki T, Murai T, Fukuda I, Tobe T, Yoshikawa M, Sasakawa C. Identification and characterization of a chromosomal virulence gene, vacJ, required for intercellular spreading of *Shigella flexneri. Mol Microbiol* 1994; 11: 31-41.
15. Bernardini ML, Mounier J, d'Hauteville H, Coquis-Rondon M, Sansonetti PJ. Identification of *icsA*, a plasmid locus of *Shigella flexneri* that governs bacterial intra and intercellular spread through interaction with F-actin. *Proc Natl Acad Sci USA* 1989; 86: 3867-71.
16. Egile C, d'Hauteville H, Parsot C, Sansonetti PJ. SopA, the outer membrane protease responsible for polar localization of IcsA in *Shigella flexneri. Mol Microbiol*; 1997. 23: 1063-73.
17. Suzuki T, Shinsuke S, Sasakawa C. Functional analysis of *Shigella* VirG domains essential for interaction with vinculin and actin-based motility. *J Biol Chem* 1996; 271: 21878-85.
18. Reinhard M, Rudiger M, Jockusch B, Walter U. VASP interaction with vinculin: a recurring theme of interactions with proline-rich motifs. *FEBS Letters* 1996; 399: 103-7.
19. Adam T, Arpin M, Prévost MC, Gounon P, Sansonetti PJ. Cytoskeletal rearrangements and the functional role of T-plastin during entry of *Shigella flexneri* into HeLa cells. *J Cell Biol* 1995; 129: 367-81.
20. Nobes CD, Hall A. Rho, Rac and Cdc42 GTPases regulate the assembly of multimolecular focal complexes associated with actin stress fibers, lamellipodia, and filopodia. *Cell* 1995; 81: 53-62.
21. Adam T, Giry M, Boquet P, Sansonetti P. Rho-dependent membrane folding causes *Shigella* entry into epithelial cells. *EMBO J* 1996; 15: 3315-21.
22. Dehio C, Prévost MC, Sansonetti PJ. Invasion of epithelial cells by *Shigella flexneri* induces tyrosine phosphorylation of cortactin by a $pp60^{c\text{-}src}$ mediated signalling pathway. *EMBO J* 1995; 14: 2471-82.

23. Isberg RR. Discrimination between intracellular uptake and surface adhesion of bacterial pathogens. *Science* 1991; 252: 934-8.
24. Rosqvist R, Håkansson S, Forsberg A, Wolf-Watz H. Functional conservation of the secretion and translocation machinery for virulence proteins of *Yersinia, Salmonellae* and *Shigellae*. *EMBO J* 1995; 14: 4187-95.

Recent advances in the pathogenesis of gastrointestinal bacterial infections.
P. Rampal, P. Boquet, eds. John Libbey Eurotext, Paris © 1998, pp. 97-109.

Yersinia enterocolitica, a very sophisticated pathogen in our everyday life

Guy R. Cornelis

Microbial Pathogenesis Unit, Christian de Duve Institute of Cellular Pathology and Université catholique de Louvain, UCL 74-49, B-1200 Brussels, Belgium

The *Yersinia* life style

For a long time, it was commonly held that each invasive pathogenic bacterium has its own life style, and that there is a great diversity of individual bacterial virulence strategies. However, recent data from several laboratories challenge this view and reveal the existence of related major virulence systems in various pathogenic bacteria, including phytopathogens. One of these systems involves the delivery of bacterial proteins inside eukaryotic cells by surface-bound bacteria that are in close contact with the target cell surface. The Yop virulon of *Yersiniae* represents the archetype of this growing family of systems.

The genus *Yersinia* includes three species that are pathogenic for rodents and humans: *Y. pestis* is the agent of black death, *Y. pseudotuberculosis* causes adenitis and septicemia and *Y. enterocolitica*, the most prevalent in humans, causes a broad range of gastrointestinal syndromes. In spite of differences in the infection routes, they share a common tropism for lymphoid tissues and a common capacity to resist the non-specific immune response. Anatomo-pathological examinations of artificially-infected mice show that *Yersinia* form extracellular microcolonies. In accordance with these *in vivo* observations, *Yersinia* are resistant to phagocytosis *in vitro*, by macrophages and polymorphonuclear leukocytes. Once they are phagocytosed, *Y. pseudotuberculosis* and *Y. enterocolitica* are generally killed.

The clue: calcium dependency

It has been known since the mid fifties that *Y. pestis* does not grow at 37° C in Ca^{2+}-deprived media. Since the loss of this unusual property correlates with a loss of virulence, non-virulent mutants could easily be detected and even selected for. Both phenotypes are determined by a 70-kb plasmid (pYV), which *in vitro* governs the massive release of a set of about 12 proteins called Yops. Genetic analyses revealed that these Yops are essential for virulence but three observations were disturbing: (i) Yops are not produced in the presence of the mM concentrations of Ca^{2+} that prevail in the extracellular fluid; (ii) *in vitro*, Yops have no obvious toxic activity on their own; and (iii) Yops form large and insoluble aggregates in the culture medium.

From the enigma to a model

Rosqvist *et al.* [1] first showed that extracellular adherent Yersinia induce a cytotoxic effect on HeLa cells and that YopE is involved in this action. However, crude preparations containing YopE had no cytotoxic effect unless they were microinjected into HeLa cells, indicating that the target of YopE is intracellular. A *yopD* mutant was also unable to affect HeLa cells but a preparation of Yops secreted by this mutant was cytotoxic when microinjected into the cytosol of HeLa cells. They concluded from this that YopD plays a role in translocating YopE across the plasma membrane of the target cell to reach the cytosolic compartment. They also showed that intracellular bacteria are not cytotoxic, which ruled out that YopE is translocated across the membrane of a phagosome. The evidence for YopD-mediated translocation of YopE was confirmed by two independent approaches. One used immunofluorescence and confocal laser scanning microscopy to show that YopE appeared in the perinuclear region of HeLa cells infected with wild-type *Y. pseudotuberculosis*. However, when infection was carried out with a *yopD* mutant, YopE was only found in spots in the vicinity of bacteria adhering to the cell surface [2]. The other approach was based on a reporter enzyme strategy, introduced by our laboratory. The reporter consisted of the calmodulin-activated adenylate cyclase domain (Cya) of the *Bordetella pertussis* cyclolysin. Since the catalytic domain of cyclolysin is unable to enter eukaryotic cells by itself, accumulation of cAMP reflects Yop internalization. Infection of HeLa cells with *Y. enterocolitica* producing a hybrid YopE-Cya resulted in a marked increase in cAMP, even when internalization of the bacteria themselves was prevented by cytochalasin D. Infection with a *yopBD* mutant did not lead to cAMP accumulation, confirming the involvement of YopD and/or YopB in translocation of YopE across eukaryotic membranes [3].

A coherent picture emerged from these two approaches: the Yops form two distinct groups of proteins: some, like YopE, are effectors that are delivered inside eukaryotic cells by extracellular yersinia, while YopB, YopD and possibly other Yops form a delivery apparatus. Both groups of proteins are secreted by the same specialized secretion system. The pYV plasmid thus encodes an integrated anti-host system that we call the Yop virulon. For the rest of this review, we will call "secretion" the crossing of the two bacterial lipid membranes and "translocation" the crossing of the eukaryotic cell plasma membrane. Yops involved in translocation of effectors will be referred to as "translocators".

Intracellular effectors

Six Yop effectors have been formally identified: YopE, YopH, YopO/YpkA, YopM, YopP and YopT.

The 23-kDa YopE causes disruption of the actin microfilament structure of cultured HeLa cells. However, it does not disrupt actin filaments polymerized *in vitro*, even in the presence of NAD^+, suggesting that its action is indirect. The target of YopE is still unknown, but it is interesting to note that YopE shares homology with Exoenzyme S of *Pseudomonas aeruginosa* that was recently shown to be secreted by a contact secretion pathway [4] and which elicits the same cytotoxicity as YopE when injected by a recombinant *Y. pseudotuberculosis* [5]. This may indicate that the two proteins have the same target(s). Since ExoS modifies small G-proteins involved in the regulation of the actin network, (see [6] for a recent review) it is possible that the effect of YopE is also mediated by some modification of small G-proteins.

YopH is a 51-kDa, broad-spectrum protein tyrosine phosphatase related to eukaryotic PTPases. Though the catalytic domain is only ~ 20% identical to human PTP1B, the Yersinia PTPase contains all of the invariant residues present in eukaryotic PTPases and forming the phosphate-binding loop (P-loop) including the nucleophilic Cys403 which forms a phosphocysteine intermediate during catalysis [7]. It acts on macrophages tyrosine-phosphorylated proteins [8], which contributes to the inhibition of bacterial uptake [8] and oxidative burst [9], presumably by dephosphorylating key proteins involved in signal transduction. YopH also obstructs the invasin stimulated uptake of Yersinia by HeLa cells. This uptake is associated with increased tyrosine phosphorylation and recruitment to peripheral complexes of $p130^{Cas}$ and FAK, two proteins that are dephosphorylated by YopH [10, 11].

YpkA is an 81-kDa serine/threonine kinase that shows noticeable sequence similarity to eukaryotic counterparts [12]. It is targeted to the inner surface of the plasma membrane of the eukaryotic cell [13]. Given the kinase activity of YpkA and its spatial localization it is reasonable to suggest that YpkA also interferes with some signal transduction pathway of the eukaryotic cell.

YopM is an acidic 41-kDa protein that contains a succession of 12 repeated structures [14] related to the very common leucine rich repeat (LRR) motifs [15]. Because of these LRR motifs, YopM exhibits a weak similarity with a large number of proteins, among which many proteoglycans. The intracellular role of yopM remains unknown.

The 30-Kda YopP induces apoptosis in macrophages by a mechanism that is not yet understood [16]. YopP is also involved [17] in the Yersinia induced suppression of TNFα release by macrophages [18], a suppression that is accompanied by the inhibition of the activity of the ERK1/2, p38 and JNK mitogen-activated protein kinases (MAPK) [19]. Whether this suppression is a consequence of apoptosis or an independent event is not yet known. Interestingly, YopP (and YopJ) share a high level of similarity with AvrRxv from *Xanthomonas campestris*. AvrRxv is one of many avirulence proteins identified in plant pathogenic bacteria that mediate the hypersensitive response, a process that results from the activation of a programmed cell death pathway. The hypersensitive response of plants requires a functional type III secretion apparatus (related to the *Yersinia* Ysc secretion apparatus) and it is generally believed that it results from the delivery of avirulence proteins into the cytosol of the plant cell [20]. YopP is thus related to a protein that is presumably an effector delivered by a plant pathogen into the cells of its host. In conclusion, YopP is a fifth Yop effector and its similarity to an effector of a plant pathogen is particularly fascinating.

Finally, YopT is a new cytotoxic effector of 35.5 kDa that effects the cytoskeleton of the eukaryotic cell by disrupting the actin filaments (Iriarte and Cornelis, in preparation).

The delivery apparatus

YopD is the first element of the delivery apparatus that was identified [2, 3, 21]. It is encoded, together with two other Yops -LcrV and YopB- by the large *lcrGVHyopBD* operon. Recent analysis of non polar *yopB* and *yopD* mutants showed that YopB is also individually required for translocation of the effectors across the eukaryotic cell plasma membrane [13, 22]. Further study on YopB showed that it causes a hemolysis of erythrocytes and that this lysis can be blocked by the addition of dextran but not raffinose [23]. These results suggest that YopB forms a pore through which the Yop-effectors are likely to be translocated. This pore-formation has not been studied *in vitro* yet.

LcrV and LcrG are also required for translocation. Using a non-polar lcrV mutant, we observed that LcrV is required for the secretion of YopB and YopD [24]. In agreement with this, we observed that LcrV binds to YopB and to YopD [24]. Taking into account that gene *sycD* encodes a chaperone for YopB and YopD (see below), the whole *lcrGVsycDyopBD* operon is thus devoted to the translocation process.

Close contact requirement

One could argue that Yops resemble exotoxins like cholera or pertussis toxin which are usually composed of two functionally distinct subunits: a toxic moiety (subunit A) and a vector (subunit B). Yops could simply be a mixture of proteins of the A and B types and various A proteins would be translocated by a complex vector made of various B proteins. Three experimental arguments support the idea that Yops are different from A-B exotoxins. First, different bacteria-free preparations of Yops, free from bacteria do not mediate any biological effect if added to cultured cells but they do induce a cytotoxic effect when they are artificially introduced into these cells. This contrasts with exotoxins which execute their activity when simply added to cultured eukaryotic cells. The second argument is the requirement for the adherence of bacteria to their target cell [2, 3]. The third argument is the absence of translocation of effectors when HeLa cells are co-infected with pairs of yersinia: one producing the effector and the second the translocators and adhesins [2, 25].

In conclusion, translocation of effector Yops is achieved by extracellular bacteria adhering at the cells surface.

Control of Yop release

Delivery of Yops into eukaryotic cells is oriented, in the sense that it occurs on the side of the bacterium which is in contact with the eukaryotic cell. The actual signal triggering Yop secretion *in vivo* would thus be contact with a eukaryotic cell. Such a contact needs to involve both a eukaryotic and a bacterial receptor. The former has not been identified yet but there are two candidates for the interactive partner on the bacterium: YopN and TyeA. Indeed, *yopN* and *tyeA* mutants release large amounts of Yops into the eukaryotic cell culture medium. While *yopN* mutants still inject Yops into the eukaryotic cells [2, 26, 22], *tyeA* mutants can no longer deliver YopE and YopH but they still deliver the four other effectors [27]. YopN and Tye thus represent two elements controlling the deployment of the translocation apparatus and the release of effectors. They presumably form a complex stop-valve, anchored to the most external part of the secretion apparatus. TyeA binds also to YopD, which is in good agreement with the requirement of LcrG for translocation [27].

lcrG mutants also release large amounts of Yops into the medium but, at variance with *yopN* mutants, they are unable to translocate the effectors (Sarker *et al.*, in preparation). LcrG could thus also be involved in the control of Yops release. We observed recently that LcrG binds to heparan sulfate. Moreover, addition of exogenous heparin decreases the level of YopE-Cya translocation into HeLa cells, suggesting that heparan sulfate proteoglycans may act as receptors at the surface of HeLa cells [28]. However, heparin has no effect on Yop secretion *in vitro*. These experiments reinforce the assumption that LcrG is part of the recognition complex at the bacterial surface but it must be stressed that, up till now, we could not gain direct evidence for a surface location of LcrG.

The Ysc secretion pathway

Effector and translocator Yops are transported across the two bacterial membranes and the bacterial cell wall by a specialized secretion system that represents the first recognized member of the "type III" family of secretion systems [29]. The secretion apparatus is encoded by about 20 genes clustered in three operons of the pYV plasmid called *virA (lcrA)*, *virB (lcrB)* and *virC (lcrC)* [30-35].

Only a few of these gene products have been characterized so far. Locus *virA* encodes the LcrD protein, an inner membrane protein with eight membrane-spanning domains and a cytoplasmic C-terminal tail [31]. Locus *virB*, comprising the eight *yscN-yscU* genes, encodes at least two other inner membrane proteins (YscR and YscU) and an ATP-binding protein called YscN [32-34, 36]. Among the thirteen *virC* gene products, there is an outer membrane protein (YscC), a lipoprotein (YscJ), and a secreted Yop (YopR, the *yscH* gene product) [30, 35, 37]. The outer membrane protein YscC forms very stable ring-shaped multimers of about 200 Å with a central pore [38]. It has homologues not only in other type III secretion systems but also in the main terminal branch of the general secretory pathway and in the extrusion system of the filamentous phages (protein PIV). The proper targeting of YscC to the outer membrane requires a lipoprotein called VirG [35, 38]. Since VirG belongs to the secretion apparatus, a more appropriate designation might be the YscW protein. Gene *virG* is localized between the *virB* and *virC* operons, close to the *virF* gene.

Some of the products encoded by the *virA* and *virC* operons behave as Yops, in the sense that they are released when Ca^{2+} ions are chelated. In particular, the *virA* operon encodes not only the LcrD protein (inner membrane) but also the YopN sensor (see above). Similarly, the *virC* operon encodes the YopR protein [35]. This raises some questions about the independence of the secretion and delivery systems and suggests that both systems are intimately coupled at the bacterial surface.

Homologues of the Ysc proteins, as well as of the LcrD protein have been identified in the flagellum secretion and assembly apparatus [39], suggesting that the Yop secretion and delivery systems might have evolved from that involved in flagellum biogenesis. Thus yersiniae, which are motile bacteria, possess two closely related secretion machineries [40]. Simultaneous expression of both probably needs to be prevented by appropriate switches. Not surprisingly, production of flagella only occurs below 30° C and requires sigma-28 factor of the RNA polymerase, whereas Yop secretion only occurs at 37° C, independently of sigma factor 28 [41, 40].

Modular structure of the Yop effectors

The signal required to secrete a Yop is located in the N-terminal region of the protein but it does not have the features of a classical signal peptide and it is not cleaved off during secretion [25] showed that this signal is contained within the 15 and 17 first residues of YopE and YopH, respectively. The effector Yops that are internalized must also be recognized by the translocation apparatus. To define the putative translocation signal on YopE and YopH [25] engineered a panoply of *yop-cya* hybrid genes by gradual deletions. Internalization into cultured macrophages only required the 50 N-terminal amino acid residues of YopE and 71 N-terminal residues of YopH. YopE and YopH are thus modular proteins composed of a secretion domain, a translocation domain and an effector domain [25] *(figure 1)*. The same applies to YopM [22].

The Syc cytosolic body guards

Secretion of YopE and YopH requires individual cytosolic chaperones called "Syc" for "Specific Yop chaperone" [42]. The Syc proteins specifically bind their cognate Yop partner in the bacterial cytoplasm. There is only one Syc-binding domain on YopE and YopH and this site corresponds exactly to the translocation site that we have defined before [43]. Interestingly, YopH and YopE derivatives deprived of the Syc-binding site maintain a normal secretion level, even in *sycE* mutants, indicating that it is the binding domain that makes the Syc chaperone necessary for Yop secretion [43]. SycH and SycE could thus act as anti-association factors, a role reminescent of that of PapD which caps the pilin subunits in the periplasm and, in doing so, impedes nonproductive interactions [44]. Since the SycE and SycH binding domains match the domains required for translocation of YopE and YopH across eukaryotic cell membranes, the chaperones probably prevent intrabacterial interaction between the effectors YopE and YopH and elements of the translocation apparatus.

The SycD chaperone appears to be slightly different from the SycE and SycH chaperones in that it protects more than one Yop: SycD binds not only the YopD translocator [45] but also the YopB translocator (Neyt and Cornelis, in preparation). Since YopB and YopD are both required for translocation of all the effectors, they are likely to associate in order to build the delivery apparatus. One hypothesis might be that the SycD chaperone prevents the intrabacterial association of the YopB and YopD translocators. This role is very reminiscent of the IpgC protein from *Shigella flexneri* that prevents premature oligomerization of the IpaB and IpaC proteins [46]. However, SycD could also cap YopD and YopB in the bacterial cytosol, in order to reduce the toxicity due to their hydrophobicity (Neyt and Cornelis, in preparation).

The three Syc proteins are dissimilar in terms of amino acid sequence but they share a few common properties, namely an acidic pI (around 4.5), a molecular mass in the range of 15-20 kDa, a putative amphipathic α-helix in the C-terminal portion, and the capacity to bind their cognate Yop. The SycE chaperone forms a homodimer [47].

Regulation of the system

Most if not all the genes involved in Yop synthesis and delivery are organized as a single regulon under a dual transcriptional control. The first level of regulation, which puts the genes on the alert when the temperature reaches 37° C, results from the temperature-influenced interplay between a transcriptional activator, VirF (LcrF in *Y. pestis* and *Y. pseudotuberculosis*) and chromatin structure [48, 49]. The second regulation prevents full expression of *yop* genes as long as the secretion apparatus is closed. By analogy with the secreted anti-σ factor involved in regulation of flagellum synthesis [50], the most likely hypothesis is that feedback inhibition is mediated by an inhibitor that is normally expelled *via* the Yop secretion apparatus. Genetical evidences show that the secreted LcrQ protein of *Y. pseudotuberculosis* (YscM in *Y. enterocolitica*) is involved in this negative control of *yop* gene expression but it remains to be shown if LcrQ/YscM is directly or indirectly involved in *yop* genes control [51, 52]. Hence, according to the model, upregulation of *yop* expression and polarized translocation of Yop-effectors are triggered by the opening of the secretion apparatus in response to the signal generated upon interaction of the pathogen with its target cell.

An evolutionary observation

The system described here above is highly conserved in *Y. enterocolitica*, *Y. pestis* and *Y. pseudotuberculosis*: most of the elements have been characterized in the three species and no significant differences have been identified. Although the genes are very conserved, the pYV plasmid in the three species suffered some reshuffling. On completion of the nucleotide sequence analysis of the *Y. enterocolitica* O:9 pYV plasmid, a potentially interesting evolutionary clue was revealed. Genes encoding Yop synthesis and secretion are tightly clustered in three quadrants of the pYV plasmid, while the fourth quadrant contains a class II transposon that confers arsenite and arsenate resistance [53] *(figure 1)*. The *ars* operon is present in the pYV plasmids of all the low virulence *Y. enterocolitica* strains tested. It was not detected in the pYV plasmid of the more virulent American strains of *Y. enterocolitica* and in the pYV plasmids from *Y. pseudotuberculosis* and *Y. pestis* [53]. This suggests that the low virulence strains, which are distributed worldwide, constitute a single phylum that probably emerged more recently. One may wonder whether the acquisition of the *ars* genes coincided with the conquest of a new ecological habitat that ensured the recent worldwide spread of these low virulence strains. At the present time, pigs represent the major reservoir of pathogenic strains of *Y. enterocolitica* and contaminated pork meat is recognized as the major human source of contamination [54]. One may, thus, wonder whether the *ars* transposon favoured the settling of a strain of *Y. enterocolitica* in pigs. In this regard, one should remember that arsenic compounds were largely used before World War II as therapeutic agents to treat pigs infected with *Serpulina hyodysenteriae*.

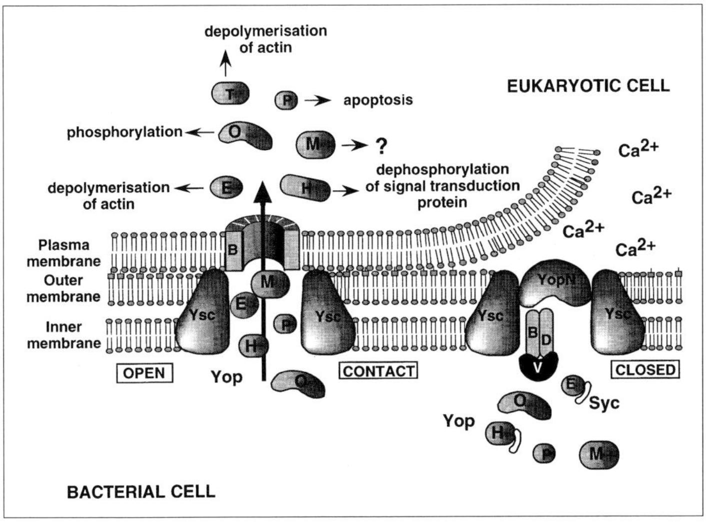

Figure 1. A model summarizing the interaction between *Yersinia* and eukaryotic target cell. As long as there is no contact with a eukaryotic cell (right), the YopN+LcrG stop-valve blocks the Ysc secretion channel. No Yops are secreted. Upon contact with the eukaryotic target cell, a sensor (YopN?, TyeA?, LcrG?) interacts with some receptor on the cell surface (proteoglycan?), which results in the opening of the secretion channel at the zone of contact. During their intrabacterial stage, Yops are capped with their specific chaperone, presumably to prevent premature associations. The Yops are then transported through the secretion channels and the Yop effectors are translocated across the plasma membrane guided by YopB and YopD.

Prospects

The Yop virulon constitutes a new and sophisticated type of bacterial weapon *(figure 1)*. Although broader details of the underlying mechanisms are now understood, many interesting questions remain regarding the Ysc secretion apparatus and the exact structure of the delivery apparatus. The role of the effectors is no less fascinating: the study of the exact role of this fifth column would lead to a better understanding of the cellular processes that are sabotaged. Since the Yop virulon appears to be the archetype of a family of related systems encountered in other pathogenic Gram negative bacteria (for recent reviews, see [55, 56], it is of broad interest. Its understanding might allow the development of a new class of antibacterial agents designed to inhibit the deployment of the virulon rather than to kill bacteria. Finally, the system also has interesting laboratory applications: *Yersinia* possessing the secretion/translocation apparatus but devoid of effectors could be engineered to introduce various proteins into eukaryotic cells. The efficacy of the system is illustrated by translocation of the adenylate cyclase.

Summary

The Yop virulon enables Yersiniae (Yersinia pestis, Y. pseudotuberculosis *and* Y. enterocolitica) *to survive and multiply in the lymphoid tissues of their host. It is an integrated system allowing extracellular bacteria to communicate with the host cell's cytosol by the injection of effector proteins. It is composed of four elements: i) a contact or type III secretion system called Ysc, devoted to the secretion of Yop proteins. This secretion apparatus, made of some 22 proteins recognizes the Yops by a short N-terminal signal that is not cleaved off during secretion; ii) a system designed to deliver bacterial proteins into eukaryotic target cells. This system involves YopB, YopD, LcrG and LcrV; iii) a control element (YopN, TyeA) and iv) a set of effector Yop proteins designed to disarm these cells or disrupt their communications (YopE, YopH, YopM, YpkA/YopO, YopP/YopJ, YopT). The whole virulon is encoded by a 70-kb plasmid called pYV.*

References

1. Rosqvist R, Forsberg A, Wolf Watz H. Intracellular targeting of the *Yersinia* YopE cytotoxin in mammalian cells induces actin microfilament disruption. *Infect Immun* 1991; 59: 4562-9.
2. Rosqvist R, Magnusson KE, Wolf Watz H. Target cell contact triggers expression and polarized transfer of *Yersinia* YopE cytotoxin into mammalian cells. *EMBO J* 1994; 13: 964-72.
3. Sory MP, Cornelis GR. Translocation of a hybrid YopE-adenylate cyclase from *Yersinia enterocolitica* into HeLa cells. *Mol Microbiol* 1994; 14: 583-94.
4. Yahr TL, Goranson J, Frank DW. Exoenzyme S of *Pseudomonas aeruginosa* secreted by a type III secretion pathway. *Mol Microbiol* 1996; 22: 991-1003.
5. Frithz-Lindsten E, Du Y, Rosqvist R, Forsberg A. Intracellular targeting of exoenzyme S of *Pseudomonas aeruginosa via* type III-dependent translocation induces phagocytosis resistance, cytotoxicity and disruption of actin microfilaments. *Mol Microbiol* 1997; 25: 1125-39.
6. Goranson J, Frank DW. Genetic analysis of exoenzyme S expression by *Pseudomonas aeruginosa*. *FEMS Microbiol Letts* 1996; 135: 149-55.
7. Stuckey JA, Schubert HL, Fauman EB, Zhang ZY, Dixon JE, Saper MA. Crystal structure of *Yersinia* protein tyrosine phosphatase at 2.5 A and the complex with tungstate. *Nature* 1994; 370: 571-5.
8. Andersson K, Carballeira N, Magnusson KE, Persson C, Stendahl O, Wolf-Watz H, Fällman M. YopH of *Yersinia pseudotuberculosis* interrupts early phosphotyrosine signalling associated with phagocytosis. *Mol Microbiol* 1996; 20: 1057-69.
9. Bliska JB, Black DS. Inhibition of the Fc receptor-mediated oxidative burst in macrophages by the *Yersinia pseudotuberculosis* tyrosine phosphatase. *Infect Immun* 1995; 63: 681-5.
10. Persson C, Carballeira N, Wolf-Watz H, Fällman M. The PTPase YopH inhibits uptake of *Yersinia*, tyrosine phosphorylation of $p130^{Cas}$ and FAK, and the associated accumulation of these proteins in peripheral focal adhesions. *EMBO J* 1997; 16: 2307-18.
11. Black DS, Bliska JB. Identification of $p130^{Cas}$ as a substrate of *Yersinia* YopH (Yop51), a bacterial protein tyrosine phosphatase that translocates into mammalian cells and targets focal adhesions. *EMBO J* 1997; 16: 2730-44.
12. Galyov EE, Hakansson S, Forsberg A, Wolf-Watz H. A secreted protein kinase of *Yersinia pseudotuberculosis* is an indispensable virulence determinant. *Nature* 1993; 361: 730-2.
13. Hakansson S, Galyov EE, Rosqvist R, Wolf-Watz H. The *Yersinia* YpkA Ser/Thr kinase is translocated and subsequently targeted to the inner surface of the HeLa cell plasma membrane. *Mol Microbiol* 1996; 20: 593-603.
14. Leung KY, Straley SC. The *yopM* gene of *Yersinia pestis* encodes a released protein having homology with the human platelet surface protein GPIb α. *J Bacteriol* 1989; 171: 4623-32.
15. Kobe B, Deisenhofer J. The leucine-rich repeat: a versatile binding motif. *TIBS* 1994; 19: 415-20.

16. Mills SD, Boland A, Sory MP, *et al. Yersinia enterocolitica* induces apoptosis in macrophages by a process requiring functional type III secretion and translocation mechanisms and involving YopP, presumably acting as an effector protein. *Proc Natl Acad Sci USA* 1997; 94: 12638-43.
17. Boland A, Cornelis GR. Suppression of macrophage TNFα release during *Yersinia* infection: role of YopP. *Infect Immun* 1998; in press.
18. Nakajima R, Brubaker RR. Association between virulence of *Yersinia pestis* and suppression of gamma interferon and tumor necrosis factor alpha. *Infect Immun* 1993; 61: 23-31.
19. Ruckdeschel K, Machold J, Roggenkamps A, *et al. Yersinia enterocolitica* promotes deactivation of macrophage mitogen-activated protein kinases extracellular signal-regulated kinase-1/2, p38, and c-Jun NH_2-terminal kinase. *J Biol Chem* 1997; 272: 15920-7.
20. Van den Acherveken G, Marois E, Bonas U. Recognition of the bacterial avirulence protein AvrBs3 occurs inside the host plant cell. *Cell* 1996; 87: 1307-16.
21. Hartland EL, Green SP, Phillips WA, Robins Browne RM. Essential role of YopD in inhibition of the respiratory burst of macrophages by *Yersinia enterocolitica. Infect Immun* 1994; 62: 4445-53.
22. Boland A, Sory MP, Iriarte M, Kerbourch C, Wattiau P, Cornelis GR. Status of YopM and YopN in the *Yersinia* Yop virulon: YopM of *Y. enterocolitica* is internalized inside the cytosol of PU5-1.8 macrophages by the YopB, D, N delivery apparatus. *EMBO J* 1996; 15: 5191-201.
23. Hakansson S, Schesser K, Persson C, Galyov EE, Roswvist R, Homble F, Wolf-Watz H. The YopB protein of *Yersinia pseudotuberculosis* is essential for the translocation of Yop effector proteins across the target cell plasma membrane and displays a contact dependent membrane disrupting activity. *EMBO* 1996; 15: 5812-23.
24. Sarker MR, Neyt C, Stainier I, Cornelis GR. The *Yersinia* Yop virulon: LcrV is required for extrusion of the translocators YopB and YopD. *J Bacteriol* 1998; 180: in press.
25. Sory MP, Boland A, Lambermont I, Cornelis GR. Identification of the YopE and YopH domains required for secretion and internalization into the cytosol of macrophages, using the *cyaA* gene fusion approach. *Proc Natl Acad Sci USA* 1995; 92: 11998-2002.
26. Persson C, Nordfelth R, Holmstr"m A, Hakansson S, Rosqvist R, Wolf-Watz H. Cell-surface-bound *Yersinia* translocate the protein tyrosine phosphatase YopH by a polarized mechanism into the target cell. *Mol Microbiol* 1995; 18: 135-50.
27. Iriarte M, Sory MP, Boland A, Boyd AP, Mills SD, Lambermont I, Cornelis GR. TyeA, a protein involved in control of Yop release and in translocation of *Yersinisa* Yop effectors. *EMBO J* 1998; in press.
28. Boyd AP, Sory MP, Iriarte M, Cornelis GR. Heparin interferes with translocation of Yop proteins into HeLa cells and binds to LcrG, a regulatory component of the *Yersinia* Yop apparatus. *Mol Microbiol* 1998; 27: 425-36.
29. Michiels T, Wattiau P, Brasseur R, Ruysschaert JM, Cornelis G. Secretion of Yop proteins by *Yersiniae*. *Infect Immun* 1990; 58: 2840-9.
30. Michiels T, Vanooteghem JC, Lambert de Rouvroit C, *et al.* Analysis of *virC*, an operon involved in the secretion of Yop proteins by *Yersinia enterocolitica. J Bacteriol* 1991; 173: 4994-5009.
31. Plano GV, Straley SC. Multiple effects of *lcrD* mutations in *Yersinia pestis. J Bacteriol* 1993; 175: 3536-45.
32. Bergman T, Erickson K, Galyov E, Persson C, Wolf Watz H. The *lcrB (yscN/U)* gene cluster of *Yersinia pseudotuberculosis* is involved in Yop secretion and shows high homology to the *spa* gene clusters of *Shigella flexneri* and Salmonella typhimurium. *J Bacteriol* 1994; 176: 2619-26.
33. Fields KA, Plano GV, Straley SC. A low-$Ca2^{+}$ response (LCR) secretion *(ysc) locus lies within the lcrB* region of the LCR plasmid in *Yersinia pestis. J Bacteriol* 1994; 176: 569-79.

34. Allaoui A, Woestyn S, Sluiters C, Cornelis GR. YscU, a *Yersinia enterocolitica* inner membrane protein involved in Yop secretion. *J Bacteriol* 1994; 176: 4534-42.
35. Allaoui A, Schulte R, Cornelis GR. Mutational analysis of the *Yersinia enterocoliticia virC* operon: characterization of *yscE, F, G, I, J, K* required for Yop secretion and *yscH* encoding YopR. *Mol Microbiol* 1995; 18: 343-55.
36. Woestyn S, Allaoui A, Wattiau P, Cornelis GR. YscN, the putative energizer of the *Yersinia* Yop secretion machinery. *J Bacteriol* 1994; 176: 1561-9.
37. Rimpilainen M, Forsberg A, Wolf Watz H. A novel protein, LcrQ, involved in the low-calcium response of *Yersinia pseudotuberculosis* shows extensive homology to YopH. *J Bacteriol* 1992; 174: 3355-63.
38. Koster M, Bitter W, de Cock H, Allaoui A, Cornelis GR, Tommassen J. The outer membrane component, YscC, of the Yop secretion machinery of *Yersinia enterocolitica* forms a ring-shaped multimeric complex. *Mol Microbiol* 1997; 26: 789-98.
39. Albertini AM, Caramori T, Crabb WD, Scoffone F, Galizzi A. The *flaA* locus of *Bacillus subtilis* is part of a large operon coding for flagellar structures, motility functions, and an ATPase-like polypeptide. *J Bacteriol* 1991; 173: 3573-9.
40. Kapatral V, Minnich SA. Co-ordinate, temperature-sensitive regulation of the three *Yersinia enterocolitica* flagellin genes. *Mol Microbiol* 1995; 17: 49-56.
41. Iriarte M, Stainier I, Mikulskis AV, Cornelis GR. The *fliA* gene encoding σ 28 in *Yersinia enterocolitica. J Bacteriol* 1995; 177: 2299-304.
42. Wattiau P, Woestyn S, Cornelis GR. Customized secretion chaperones in pathogenic bacteria. *Mol Microbiol* 1996; 20: 255-62.
43. Woestyn S, Sory MP, Boland A, Lequenne O, Cornelis GR. The cytosolic SycE and SycH chaperones of *Yersinia* protect the region of YopE and YopH involved in translocation across eukaryotic cell membranes. *Mol Microbiol* 1996; 20: 1261-71.
44. Hultgren SJ, Jones CH. Utility of the immunoglobulin-like fold of chaperones in shaping organelles of attachment in pathogenic bacteria. *ASM News* 1995; 61: 457-64.
45. Wattiau P, Bernier B, Deslee P, Michiels T, Cornelis GR. Individual chaperones required for Yop secretion by *Yersinia. Proc Natl Acad Sci USA* 1994; 91: 10493-7.
46. Menard R, Sansonetti P, Parsot C, Vasselon T. Extracellular association and cytoplasmic partitioning of the IpaB and IpaC invasins of *S. flexneri. Cell* 1994; 79: 515-25.
47. Wattiau P, Cornelis GR. SycE, a chaperone-like protein of *Yersinia enterocolitica* involved in the secretion of YopE. *Mol Microbiol* 1993; 8: 123-31.
48. Cornelis GR, Sluiters C, de Rouvroit CL, Michiels T. Homology between *virF*, the transcriptional activator of the *Yersinia* virulence regulon, and AraC, the *Escherichia coli* arabinose operon regulator. *J Bacteriol* 1989; 171: 254-62.
49. Cornelis GR, Sluiters C, Delor I, Geib D, Kaniga K, Lambert de Rouvroit C, Sory MP, Vanooteghem JC, Michiels T. *ymoA*, a *Yersinia enterocolitica* chromosomal gene modulating the expression of virulence functions. *Mol Microbiol* 1991; 5: 1023-34.
50. Hughes KT, Gillen KL, Semon MJ, Karlinsey JE. Sensing structural intermediates in bacterial flagellar assembly by export of a negative regulator [see comments]. *Science* 1993; 262: 1277-80.
51. Pettersson J, Nordfelth R, Dubinina E, *et al.* Modulation of virulence factor expression by pathogen target cell contact. *Science* 1996; 273: 1231-3.
52. Stainier I, Iriarte M, Cornelis GR. YscM1 and YscM2, two *Yersinia enterocolitica* proteins causing down regulation of *yop* transcription. *Mol Microbiol* 1997; 26: 833-43.
53. Neyt C, Iriarte M, Ha Thi V, Cornelis GR. Virulence and arsenic resistance in Yersiniae. *J Bacteriol* 1997; 179: 612-9.
54. Tauxe RV, Vandepitte J, Wauters G, *et al. Yersinia enterocolitica* infections and pork: the missing link. *Lancet* 1987; ii: 1129-32.

55. Galan JE. Molecular genetic bases of *Salmonella* entry into host cells. *Mol Microbiol* 1996; 20: 263-71.
56. Menard R, Dehio C, Sansonetti PJ. Bacterial entry into epithelial cells: the paradigm of *Shigella*. *Trends Microbiol* 1996; 4: 220-5.

Recent advances in the pathogenesis of gastrointestinal bacterial infections.
P. Rampal, P. Boquet, eds. John Libbey Eurotext, Paris © 1998, pp. 111-124.

Listeria monocytogenes: strategies for entry and spread within cells and tissues

Pascale Cossart

Unité des Interactions Bactéries Cellules, Institut Pasteur, 28, rue du Docteur-Roux, Paris 75015, France

L. monocytogenes is a food borne pathogen responsible for a human disease characterized by meningitis, meningo-encephalitis, septicemias, abortions and also gastroenteritis with a mortality rate of 30%. These features are due to the very unique property of *L. monocytogenes* to be able to cross three barriers during infection: the intestinal barrier, the brain-blood barrier and/or the placental barrier.

Most of our knowledge of the human disease comes from the many studies carried out in the mouse model. The scenario of the human infection is believed to be the following: *via* contaminated food, bacteria reach the gastro-intestinal tract and cross the intestinal barrier. Recent data indicate that there is no preferential site of entry (the enterocytes or the M cells) [1]. Bacteria are subsequently engulfed by resident macrophages in which they survive and even replicate. Then, *via* the lymph and the blood, they reach the spleen and liver. In this latter organ, most of the bacteria are killed by the Kupffer cells. A fraction of the bacteria reach the hepatocytes where they induce a process of apoptosis with the concommittant release of chemoattractants which will lead to the influx of neutrophils. These phagocytic cells will ingest bacteria or apoptotic hepatocytes and contribute to the rapid clearing of the infection before the complete sterilisation by the immune response. In some cases – the immunocompromised host or the pregnant woman – bacteria multiply unrestrictedly in the hepatocytes from which they disseminate, *via* the blood, to the brain and the placenta, resulting in the characteristic clinical features of the infection described above. The key step in the establishment of a "successful" infection is the step of bacterial multiplication in the liver.

Detailed analysis of *Listeria*-infected tissue cultured cells reveals a complex series of host-pathogen interactions culminating in the direct dissemination of *L. monocytogenes* from one infected cell to another. Host cell infection begins with the internalization of the bacteria either by phagocytosis in the case of macrophages or induced phagocytosis in the case of non-phagocytic cells. Bacteria have evolved a very efficient way to enter non phagocytic cells. They push in the plasma membrane which progressively surrounds the bacterium, by a process quite different from the membrane ruffles observed during *Salmonella* or *Shigella* entry. This process is usually referred to as the "zipper" type mechanism in contrast to the "trigger" type mechanism used by *Shigella* or *Salmonella.* The bacteria are by this process very rapidly internalized within membrane-bound vacuoles where they reside during *ca* 30 min. Bacteria then lyse the vacuoles and reach the cytosol. In this environment, they start to multiply. Concommitantly, they become covered with actin filaments which within 2 h rearrange in long comet tails left behind in the cytosol while the bacteria are moving ahead at a speed of about 0.3 $\mu m\ s^{-1}$. When moving bacteria contact the plasma membrane, they induce the formation of pseudopod-like protrusions. Contact between these protrusions and neighboring cells results in the internalisation of the bacteria-containing protrusion. In the newly infected cell, the bacterium is surrounded by two plasma membranes which must be lysed to initiate a new cycle of multiplication and movement. Thus, once *Listeria* has entered the cytoplasm, it can disseminate directly from cell to cell spread circumventing such host defenses as circulating antibody and complement. This ability to disseminate in tissues by cell-to-cell spreading provides an explanation for the early observation that antibody, although induced and abundant, is not protective and that anti-*listeria* immunity is T-cell mediated.

These different phases of the infection are schematized in *figure 1.* In this figure adapted from [2], the bacterial factors involved in each specific step are indicated. Entry into mammalian cells is mediated by at least two bacterial factors: internalin (InlA) and InlB. Escape from the vacuole requires expression of listeriolysin O (LLO), a pore forming toxin which in some cells can function synergistically with or be replaced by a phosphatidylinositol-specific phospholipase C (PI-PLC). Intracellular movement requires expression of ActA, and lysis of the two-membrane vacuole is performed by a lecithinase (PlcB).

Two aspects of the infectious process will be discussed: entry into non-phagocytic mammalian cells (invasion of mammalian cells) and the actin-based motility. Several reviews have been recently published on these topics [3-5].

Invasion of mammalian cells

The *inlAB* locus

Invasion genes were identified by screening a library of Tn*1545* mutants of *L. monocytogenes* for loss of invasiness into the intestinal epithelial cell line Caco-2 [6]. Three non invasive mutants were obtained. In all three mutants, the transposon had inserted upstream from two open reading frames, *inlA* and *inlB*. Transcription of *inlA* and *inlB* was abolished in the non-invasive mutants.

The role of the first gene was demonstrated by expressing *inlA* in the non invasive bacterium *L. innocua* which became able to invade Caco-2 cells suggesting that the InlA protein may be sufficient for entry. Hence the name "internalin" given to this protein. The role of the second gene was elucidated by constructing in frame deletions in each of these two genes and testing the corresponding mutants in various cell lines [7, 8]. This approach established that InlB is also an invasion protein used for entry in some hepatocyte like cell lines, HeLa cells, Vero cells, CHO cells, revealing that the *inlAB* operon is involved in cell tropism.

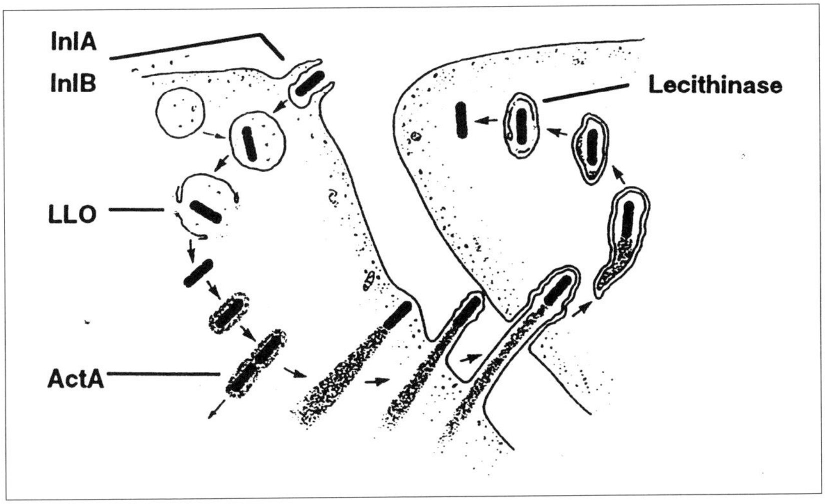

Figure 1. Schematic representation of the cell infectious process by *L. monocytogenes*. The bacterial factors involved are indicated.

Internalin, a LRR protein sufficient for entry

Internalin is an 800 amino-acid protein which displays two regions of repeats, the first being a succession of 15 twenty-two amino-acid long leucine rich repeats (LRRs) *(figure 2)*. It has the features of a protein which is targeted to and exposed on the bacterial surface, *i.e.* a signal peptide, and a C-terminal region made of a LPXTG peptide followed by a hydrophobic sequence and a few charged residues. This type of C-terminus is now found in more than 50 Gram positive bacterial surface proteins and allows a covalent linkage of the protein to the cell wall peptido-glycan, occurring after cleavage of the T-G link. Since expression of *inlA* in *L. innocua* confered invasiveness, it was anticipated that internalin could be sufficient for entry. Indeed, *inlA* when expressed in another gram positive bacterium *Enterococcus faecalis*, confers invasiveness [9]. Moreover, internalin-coated beads are invasive [9]. Internalin is thus sufficient to promote entry.

E-cadherin, the internalin receptor on epithelial cells

The internalin receptor was identified by a biochemical approach. An internalin column was used to affinity-purify the putative receptor from Caco2 extracts. After passage of the extracts on the column and extensive washings, two polypeptides were eluted by EDTA and their N-terminal sequence determined. Comparison with protein sequence data banks revealed that these two proteins were E-cadherin and its proteolytic fragment normally produced in the conditions used to prepare the extracts [10].

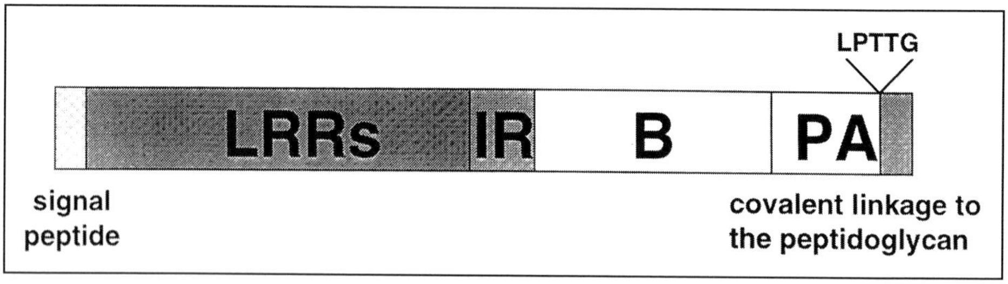

Figure 2. Schematic representation of internalin.

E-cadherin is a transmembrane glycoprotein which mediates calcium dependent cell-cell adhesion, through homophilic interactions between extracellular domains of E-cadherin. Cadherins are proteins specifically expressed in different tissues, E-cadherin in epithelial cells, N-cadherin in neuronal cells, etc. Cadherins play a critical role in cell sorting during development and in maintenance of tissue cohesion and architecture during adult life. In polarized epithelial cells, E-cadherin is mainly expressed at the adherens junctions and on the baso-lateral face. Integrity of the intracytoplasmic domain of cadherins is required for optimal intercellular adhesion. This domain interacts with proteins named catenins which in turn interact with the cytoskeleton, highlighting the importance of the cytoskeleton in maintaining adhesion of adjacent epithelial cells.

To demonstrate that the internalin-E-cadherin interaction promotes not only specific binding but also entry of *L. monocytogenes*, a set of transfected cell lines was used. Entry of both *L. monocytogenes* or *L. innocua* expressing internalin was highly promoted in cells expressing the chicken E-cadherin (L-CAM), in contrast to cells expressing N-cadherin or no cadherin. Similar results have also recently been obtained with internalin coated beads [9]. How internalin interacts with E-cadherin is under investigation. Recent data suggest that the LRRs interact directly with E-cadherin [9] but the region of E-cadherin involved in this interaction has not been identifiied yet.

Taken together, these results suggest that *in vivo*, *L. monocytogenes* does not penetrate the intestinal barrier by the apical pole of enterocytes, favoring a mechanism of translocation through M cells as a primary step in infection. Entry in enterocytes would represent a secondary step taking place at their baso-lateral face. This hypothesis is in agreement with *in vitro* observations that *Listeria* preferentially invades Caco-2 cell islets by the baso-lateral surface [11].

InlB, an invasion protein with a novel type of cell wall association

InlB is found both at the bacterial surface and to some extent in bacterial supernatants [7]. It is similar to internalin [6]. It has eight tandem leucine rich repeats (LRRs) very similar to those of internalin. It has a signal sequence but does not display the LPXTG motif or any hydrophobic region which would indicate a possible transmembrane region. Recent experiments indicate the 231 C-terminal amino-acids of InlB are necessary and sufficient to anchor this protein to the bacterial surface [12]. This region contains tandem repeats of approximately 80 amino-acids beginning with the sequence GW; similar repeats are found in a newly identified surface protein of *L. monocytogenes* named Ami and at a lesser extent in lysostaphin *(figure 3)*. Lysostaphin is a bacteriocin secreted by *Staphylococcus simulans* which associates with the cell wall of the target bacteria *S. aureus* even when added exogenously. InlB is also able when externally added to associate to *L. monocytogenes* and several other gram positive bacteria. This external association leads to entry of the Δ*inlB* mutant and also promotes entry of the non invasive species *Staphylococcus carnosus* indicating not only that InlB may interact with the cell wall after an eventual secretion or release from the bacterial surface but also that this interaction is productive for invasion [12]. The results with *S. carnosus* suggested for the first time that InlB is sufficient for entry. It has now been shown that latex beads coated with InlB enter Vero cells very efficiently [13]. In conclusion, as internalin, InlB is sufficient for entry. The InlB receptor is unknown.

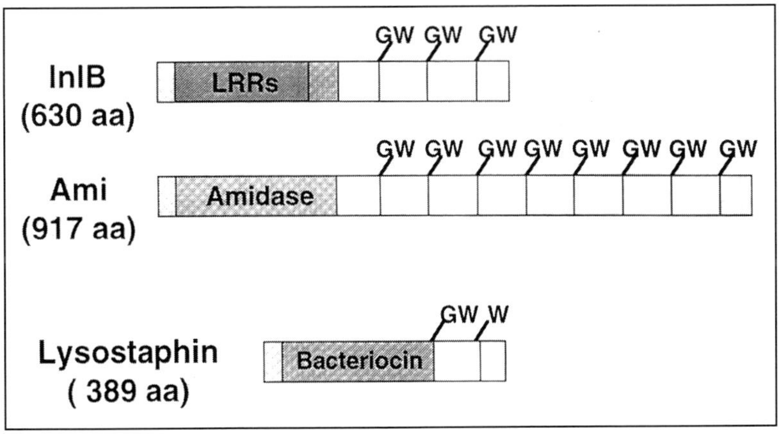

Figure 3. InlB and the GW module family.

PI 3-kinase, a signaling protein required for and activated upon entry

It was known for some time that treatment of cells with either tyrosine kinase inhibitors [14, 15] or cytochalasin D [16] inhibit entry while not inhibiting adhesion. It was thus clear that invasion requires at least one tyrosine kinase and an intact actin cytoskeleton. It has now been established that a signaling protein normally implicated in actin polymerisation in response to receptor stimulation and tyrosine phosphorylation, namely the heterodimeric lipid kinase P85/P11O PI 3-kinase, is also involved in entry of *L. monocytogenes* in mammalian cells [8].

PI-3 kinase upon receptor stimulation, migrates from the cytosol to a membrane tyrosine phosphorylated protein, *i.e.* an activated (tyrosine phosphorylated) tyrosine kinase receptor or a tyrosine-phosphorylated adaptor protein. Migration to the plasma membrane stimulates activity of PI-3 kinase, by placing the enzyme in a compartment where its substrates are located and also by conformational changes after protein protein interactions. PI 3-kinase phosphorylates the D3 position of of the inositol ring of PI, PIP and PIP2 giving rise to PI3P, PI3,4P2 and PI3,4,5P3. These last two components are virtually absent in resting cells. Their levels dramatically increase upon stimulation. They are not the substrates for phospholipases and may act as second messagers by interacting with kinases such as Akt.

Wortmannin is a fungal metabolite which can specifically inhibit PI 3-kinase. All cells when pretreated with wortmannin, become less permissive to *Listeria*, with a maximal inhibitory effect of wortmannin in Vero cells. In addition, expression of a dominant negative form of P85 also inhibits *Listeria* entry. These two types of experiments clearly establish that PI-3 kinase is required for entry [8]. Moreover, measurements of the levels of phosphoinositides reveal that bacterial entry stimulates synthesis of both PI3,4P2 and PI3,4,5P3, as shown in Vero cells. This synthesis is inhibited by pretreating cells with wortmannin, but is not by pretreatment with cytochalasin D providing evidence that cytoskeleton rearrangements occur downstream from the PI-3 kinase stimulation, during bacterial invasion. Interestingly, PI-3 kinase stimulation is inhibited by genistein. In agreement with this observation, PI-3 kinase can be, shortly after infection, co-immunoprecipitated with at least one tyrosine phosphorylated protein bringing evidence that upon entry PI-3 kinase activity is stimulated after interaction with at least one tyrosine phosphorylated protein.

A ΔinlB mutant still adheres to Vero cells but does not efficiently stimulate PI 3 kinase and does not stimulate association of PI 3 kinase with tyrosine phosphorylated proteins. Thus InlB seems to play a critical role in the stimulation of P85/P110.

How stimulation of PI3 kinase affects bacterial invasion is not known. Intriguingly, the internalin-E cadherin mediated entry in Caco-2 cells which is also affected by wortmannin does not stimulate PI-3 kinase activity. Interestingly, not only the basal levels of PI3,4P2 and PI3,4,5P3 do not increase significantly upon entry but they are already very high in uninfected Caco-2 cells. Thus in Caco-2 cells, the internalin E-cadherin pathway exploits a pre-stimulated PI-3 kinase dependent pathway.

The two pathways of entry

In summary, *Listeria* can enter by two pathways *(figure 4)*. One of them can be compared to the invasin integrin pathway of *Yersinia* in which a bacterial factor interacts with a cell adhesion molecule known to interact with the cytoskeleton [17]. Although the molecules involved are different, some functional similarity exists between the two systems such as the sensibility to tyrosine kinase inhibitors or to cytochalasin D. The other pathway is the InlB dependant pathway.

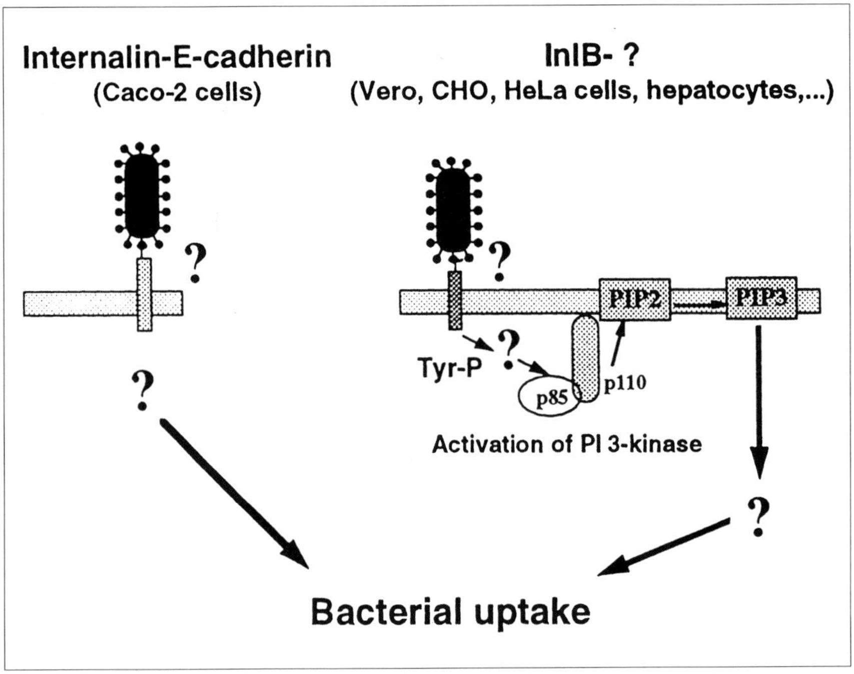

Figure 4. Schematic representation of the internalin- and InlB-mediated pathways.

The actin-based motility

This spectacular phenomenon which, by coupling actin polymerisation and movement, propels the bacteria inside the cytosol has recently received a great deal of attention since it is highly reminiscent of cellular events which remain unexplained, in particular the movement of cells such as neutrophils attracted at a site of infection, or the movement of cancer cells. It is believed that similar mechanisms could occur at the leading edge of moving cells and at the rear of the bacteria, hence the enthusiasm for a system which by its relative simplicity can be manipulated and studied more easily (for reviews, see [3-5, 18, 19]).

The relationship between the actin tail formation and movement

The early observations of thin cross sections of *Listeria*-infected cells decorated with fragment S1 of myosin revealed that the actin tails are made of cross-linked short filaments with their barbed (fast polymerizing) end oriented towards the bacterium, and suggested that actin polymerisation takes place at the rear of the bacterium. Microinjection of fluorescent actin monomers in live infected cells and video microscopy observations then demonstrated that the actin polymerisation takes place at the rear of the bacterium and that bacteria move away while the actin tail remains stationary in the cytosol. There is a strict correlation between the rate of tail formation and speed movement strongly suggesting that the force for propulsion is provided by the actin polymerisation itself.

The ActA protein

ActA was discovered by analyzing mutants which inside cells were totally unable to polymerize actin and move [20, 21]. These mutants formed microcolonies inside the cell. They were unable to spread from one cell to the other and were avirulent when injected to mice. These mutants had inactivated a gene named *actA* which encodes a protein of 610 amino-acids.

ActA has all the features of a protein which can be targeted to the bacterial surface *(figure 5)*. It has a signal sequence and a C-terminal hydrophobic region which can anchor this protein in the bacterial membrane. ActA has a polar distribution on the bacterial surface, with a higher distribution on one pole of the bacteria. In infected cells, ActA is located at the base of the actin tail suggesting that this polar distribution predetermines the site of actin assembly and the direction of movement [22].

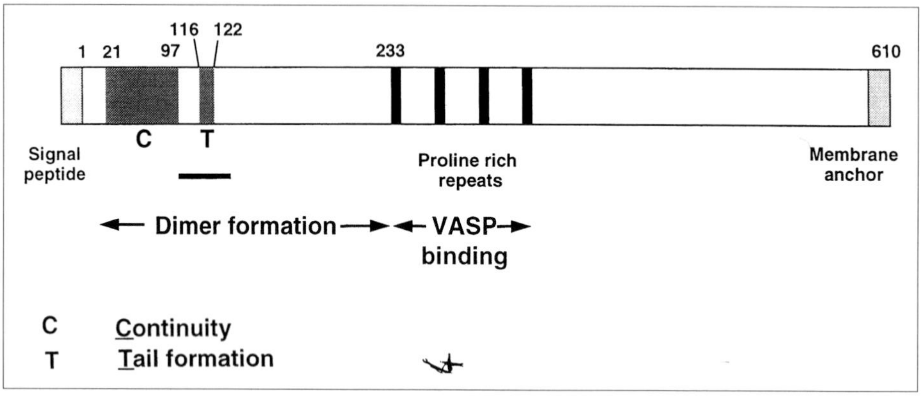

Figure 5. Critical regions in ActA.

ActA, a protein sufficient to induce actin polymerization and movement

To determine whether ActA is sufficient to induce actin polymerisation, the gene *actA* was transfected in mammalian cells where it was able to induce the polymerisation of G-actin (globular actin) into filaments (F-actin) [23, 24].

To demonstrate that ActA is not only sufficient to induce actin polymerisation but also sufficient for movement, two different experimental approaches were used:

i) production ActA in the non-pathogenic species *L. innocua* [25]: this normally non-motile bacterium became converted into an organism capable of actin polymerisation and movement in *Xenopus* cytoplasmic extracts, an *in vitro* system now commonly used to observe *listeria* movement.

ii) incubation *Steptococcus pneumoniae* with a recombinant ActA-LytA hybrid protein, which was adsorbed on and covered the streptococcal surface: the decorated bacteria became able to polymerize actin and move [26]. Interestingly, these events only occurred after bacteria had divided to generate a polar distribution of ActA on the streptococcal surface. Thus, both ActA production and its polar distribution are prerequisites for actin assembly and movement.

Homologies between ActA and other proteins

The ActA protein can be artificially divided into three parts, the N-terminal domain (1-233) which is highly charged, a central proline rich repeat region (234-395) and the C-terminal region (396-610). Recent amino-acid sequence comparisons have revealed that ActA is a composite protein. The proline-rich repeats and the carboxy-terminal domain share significant sequence similarity with zyxin, a protein associated with focal contacts and actin stress fibers [27]. The N-terminal domain of ActA is similar (25% identity) to the C-terminal region (aminoacid 879-1066) of vinculin which is a protein recently shown to be able to bind actin precisely through its C-terminal region [5]. Thus, ActA seems to have domains similar to eucaryotic proteins involved in the organization of the cytoskeleton.

The cellular factors involved

In order to address the role of ActA, the first question was: Is ActA able to bind actin? All attempts to demonstrate interactions between ActA and actin have failed, suggesting that this protein does not interact directly with actin and that at least another cellular factor is involved in the actin polymerisation process.

To identify such factors (for reviews, see [4, 5]), the main approach has been to identify proteins in the actin tails by using antibodies against known cytoskeletal proteins. Proteins identified in this way include a-actinin, tropomysosin, vinculin, villin, talin, ezrin/radixin, fimbrin, cofilin, profilin and VASP. The two most relevant proteins are profilin and VASP which colocalize with the beginning of the actin tail. VASP was shown to bind purified ActA *in vitro*, establishing the first direct link between ActA and the cytoskeleton [28]. Since VASP binds profilin, colocalization of the two proteins at the beginning of the actin tail is probably due to VASP binding to ActA [27]. This has not been demonstrated yet.

The role of some of the other proteins was assessed by different approaches. In the case of profilin, depletion of cytoplasmic extracts with polyproline beads were used. Bacterial movement was then tested in the depleted extracts. It appeared clear that most profilin can be depleted without affecting bacterial actin-based motility [29, 30]. Concerning α-actinin, microinjection of a fragment which acted as a dominant negative mutant demonstrated that this crosslinking protein is required for efficient actin tail formation and movement [31].

A very different approach was reported recently which led to the identification of other cellular factors involved in the actin-based motility [32]. Cytoplasmic extracts isolated from human platelets were fractionated and an eight polypeptide complex was purified which was sufficient to initiate ActA-dependent actin polymerisation at the surface of *L. monocytogenes*. Two subunits of this protein complex are actin-related proteins (Arps) belonging to the Arp2 and Arp3 subfamilies. The Arp3 subunit localizes to the surface of stationary bacteria and the tails of motile bacteria in *L. monocytogenes* infected tissue culture cells, consistent with a role for the complex in promoting actin assembly *in vivo*.

Genetic analysis of ActA

In order to identify the regions of ActA critical for its function, deletions in *actA* were generated which demonstrated that the N-terminal (ActAN) is absolutely critical, the central region acting as a stimulator [33, 34]. These results were confirmed by expressing in *Listeria* an ActAN-LacZ fusion which was functional for movement [34]. It was also shown by immunofluorescence using anti VASP antibodies to label infected cells, that VASP colocalizes with ActA expressing bacteria only if the central region of ActA is present, suggesting that ActA binds to the proline-rich region of ActA, a result recently confirmed by other means by Wehland and coworkers [35].

A recent analysis of the N-terminus of ActA has demonstrated that this region contains two critical regions specifically involved in actin polymerisation [33]. The first region (region T, AA 116-122) is critical for the dynamics of the process as shown by absence of a tail in a mutant with a deletion of this region. The second (region C, AA21-97) is more specifically involved in the maintenance of the continuity of the process, since deletion of this region leads to discontinuous actin tails.

Current hypothesis

Our current view of the phenomenon is that in the wild type, continuous actin-based motility occurs in three steps:

1. Generation of free barbed ends, by either nucleation, severing or uncapping.

2. Monomer addition and movement.

3. Continuous filament release/capping/cross-linking and generation of new free barbed ends.

We believe that the balance between these last two events allows continuity of the process. In the Δ21-97 mutant, free barbed ends are generated, polymerisation takes place but capping occurs more rapidly than in the wild type, so that bacteria are stalling until a critical number of free barbed ends is reached; these observations have led us to propose that ActA could play a role in protection of filament ends from capping proteins. This hypothesis implies that ActA could interact with actin, in apparent contradiction with the data mentioned above, unless one considers that ActA like vinculin has cryptic actin binding sites which need to be activated to be detectable. In fact, as we have recently shown, a peptide spanning AA 30 to 50 can bind actin.

All these considerations lead to a model presented in *figure 6* in which we have incorporated the recent information that ActA is a dimer [36]. In the model, the central part of the ActA dimer binds VASP which is a tetramer. VASP binds profilin which binds actin monomers which can be used by the N-terminal part to elongate free barbed ends. These filaments ends are protected from capping proteins by the N-terminal part of ActA. Whether Arp2 and Arp3 are recruited by the N-terminal domain of ActA or whether there is another protein involved remains to be established. It is thus possible that ActA has several functions, one of them being to protect filaments from capping proteins.

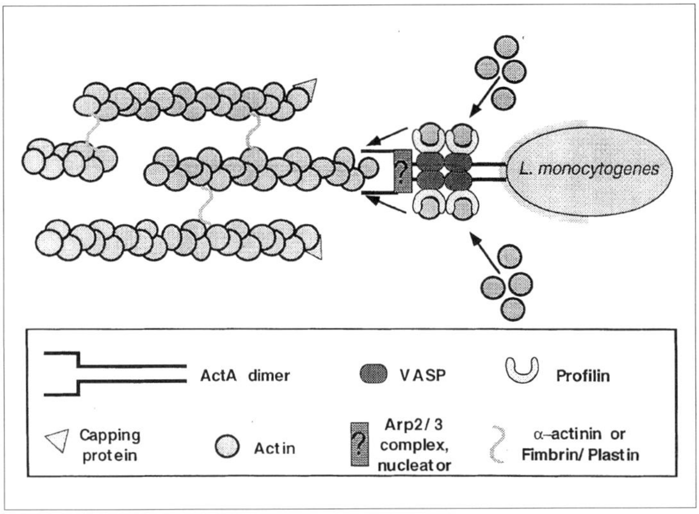

Figure 6. Model of actin assembly.

Concluding remarks

L. monocytogenes appears as an invasive bacterium which shares common features with some invasive bacteria and other features with others. For example, it enters cells by a "zipper" mechanism similar to the invasin-mediated type of entry of *Yersinia*. The later stages of the infection are more similar to those used by *Shigella* which is also internalized in a vacuole, then also escapes from this compartment and finally also spreads from cell to cell by using an actin-based motility. Interestingly, none of the genes used by *Shigella* are similar to those used by *Listeria* at simlar stages. These observations reinforce the idea that there are common themes in pathogenesis but that each bacterium has developped specific strategies to infect its host [19, 37, 38].

References

1. Pron B, Boumaila C, Jaubert F, Sarnacki S, Monnet J.P, Berche P, Gaillard JL. Comprehensive study of the intestinal stage of listeriosis in a rat ligated ileal loop system. *Infect Immun* 1998; 66: 747-755.
2. Tilney LG, Portnoy DA. Actin filaments and the growth, movement, and spread of the intracellular bacterial parasite, *Listeria monocytogenes. J Cell Biol* 1989; 109: 1597-608.
3. Cossart P. Subversion of the mammalian cytoskeleton by invasive bacteria. *J Clin Invest* 1997; 99: 2307-11.
4. Ireton K, Cossart P. Host pathogen interactions during entry and actin-based movement of *Listeria monocytogenes. Annu Rev Genet* 1997; 31: 113-38.
5. Lasa I, Dehoux P, Cossart P. Actin polymerization and bacterial movement. *Biochem Biophys Acta* 1998 (in press).
6. Gaillard JL, Berche P, Frehel C, Gouin E, Cossart P. Entry of *L. monocytogenes* into cells is mediated by internalin, a repeat protein reminiscent of surface antigens from gram-positive cocci. *Cell* 1991; 65: 1127-41.
7. Dramsi S, Biswas I, Maguin E, Braun L, Mastroeni P, Cossart P. Entry of *L. monocytogenes* into hepatocytes requires expression of InlB, a surface protein of the internalin multigene family. *Mol Microbiol* 1995; 16: 251-61.
8. Ireton K, Payrastre B, Chap H, Ogawa W, Sakaue H, Kasuga M, Cossart P. A role for phosphoinositide 3-kinase in bacterial invasion. *Science* 1996; 274: 780-2.
9. Lecuit M, Ohayon H, Braun L, Mengaud J, Cossart P. Internalin of *Listeria monocytogenes* with an intact Leucine-rich repeat region is sufficient to promote internalization. *Infect Immun* 1997; 65: 5309-19.
10. Mengaud J, Ohayon H, Gounon P, Mège RM, Cossart P. E-cadherin is the receptor for internalin, a surface protein required for entry of *Listeria monocytogenes* into epithelial cells. *Cell* 1996; 84: 923-32.
11. Gaillard JL, Finlay BB. Effect of cell polarization and differentiation on entry of *Listeria monocytogenes* into enterocyte-like Caco-2 cell line. *Infect Immun* 1996; 64: 1299-308.
12. Braun L, Dramsi S, Dehoux P, Bierne H, Lindahl G, Cossart P. InlB: an invasion protein of *Listeria monocytogenes* with a novel type of surface association. *Mol Microbiol* 1997; 25: 285-94.
13. Braun L, Ohayon H, Cossart P. The InlB protein of *Listeria monocytogenes* is sufficient to promote entry into mammalian cells. *Mol Microbiol* 1998; 27: 1077-88.
14. Velge P, Bottreau E, Kaeffer B, Yurdusev N, Pardon P, Van langendonck N. Protein tyrosine kinase inhibitors block the entries of *Listeria monocytogenes and Listeria ivanovii* into epithelial cells. *Microbiol Path* 1994; 17: 37-50.
15. Tang P, Rosenshine I, Finlay BB. *Listeria monocytogenes, an invasive bacterium, stimulates MAP kinase upon attachment to epithelials cells. Mol Biol Cell* 1994; 5: 455-64.
16. Gaillard JL, Berche P, Mounier J, Richard S, Sansonetti P. *In vitro* model of penetration and intracellular growth of *L. monocytogenes* in the human enterocyte-like cell line Caco-2. *Infect Immun* 1987; 55: 2822-9.
17. Tran Van Nhieu G, Isberg R. Bacterial internalization mediated by β_1 chain integrins is determined by ligand affinity and receptor density. *EMBO J* 1993; 12: 1887-95.
18. Cossart P. Bacterial actin based motility. *Curr Opin Cell Biol* 1995; 7: 94-101.
19. Finlay BB, Cossart P. Exploitation of mammalian host cell functions by bacterial pathogens. *Science* 1997; 276: 718-25.
20. Kocks C, Gouin E, Tabouret M, Berche P, Ohayon H, Cossart P. *Listeria monocytogenes*-induced actin assembly requires the *ActA* gene product, a surface protein. *Cell* 1992; 68: 521-31.

21. Domman E, Wehland J, Rohde M, Pistor S, Hartl M, Goebel W, Leimeister-Wächter M, Wuenscher M, Chakraborty T. A novel bacterial gene in *Listeria monocytogenes* required for host cell microfilament interaction with homology to the proline-rich region of vinculin. *EMBO J* 1992; 11: 1981-90.
22. Kocks C, Hellio R, Gounon P, Ohayon H, Cossart P. Polarized distribution of *Listeria monocytogenes* surface protein ActA at the site of directional actin assembly. *J Cell Sci* 1993; 105: 699-710.
23. Pistor S, Chakraborty T, Niebuhr K, Domann E, Wehland J. The ActA protein of *L. monocytogenes* acts as a nucleator inducing reorganization of the actin cytoskeleton. *EMBO J* 1994; 13: 758-63.
24. Friederich E, Gouin E, Hellio R, Kocks C, Cossart P, Louvard D. Targeting of *Listeria monocytogenes* ActA protein to the plasma membrane as a tool to dissect both actin-based cell morphogenesis and ActA function. *EMBO J* 1995; 14: 2731-44.
25. Kocks C, Marchand JB, Gouin E, d'Hauteville H, Sansonetti P, Carlier MF, Cossart P. The unrelated surface proteins ActA of *Listeria monocytogenes* and IcsA of *Shigella flexneri* are sufficient to confer actin-based motility to *L. innocua* and *E. coli* respectively. *Mol Microbiol* 1995; 18: 413-23.
26. Smith GA, Portnoy DA, Theriot JA. Asymmetric distribution of the *Listeria monocytogenes* ActA protein is resuired and sufficient to direct actin-based motility *Mol Microbiol* 1995; 17: 945-51.
27. Golsteyn RM, Beckerle M, Koay T, Friederich E. Structural and functional similarities between the human cytoskeletal protein zyxin and the ActA protein of *Listeria monocytogenes*. *J Cell Sci* 1997; 110: 1893-1906.
28. Chakraborty T, Ebel F, Dommann E, Niebuhr K, Gerstel B, Pistor S, Temm-Grove CJ, Jockusch BM, Reinhard M, Walter U, Wehland J. A focal adhesion factor directly linking intracellularly motile *Listeria monocytogenes* and *Listeria ivanovii* to the actin-based cytoskeleton of mammalian cells. *EMBO J* 1995; 14: 1314-21.
29. Marchand JB, Moreau P, Paoletti A, Cossart P, Carlier MF, Pantaloni D. Actin-based movement of *Listeria monocytogenes* in *Xenopus* egg extracts is due to local uncapping of the barbed ends of actin filaments at the bacterial surface and resulting shift in steady state of actin assembly. *J Cell Biol* 1995; 130: 331-43.
30. 30. Theriot JA, Rosenblatt J, Portnoy DA, Goldschmidt-Clermont PJ, Mitchison TJ. Involvement of profilin in the actin-based motility of *L. monocytogenes* in cells and in cell-free extracts. *Cell* 1994; 76: 505-17.
31. Dold FG, Sanger JM, Sanger JW. Intact alpha-actinin molecules are needed for both the assembly of actin into tails and the locomotion of *Listeria monocytogenes* inside infected cells. *Cell Mot Cytoskel* 1994; 28: 97-107.
32. Welch MD, Iwamatsu A, Mitchison TJ. Actin polymerization is induced by Arp2/3 protein complex at the surface of *Listeria monocytogenes*. *Nature* 1997; 385: 265-9.
33. Lasa I, David V, Gouin E, Marchand J, Cossart P. The amino-terminal part of ActA is critical for the actin based motility of *Listeria monocytogenes*; the central proline-rich region acts as a stimulator. *Mol Microbiol* 1995; 18: 425-36.
34. Lasa I, Gouin E, Goethals M, Vancompernolle K, David V, Vandekerckhove J, Cossart P. Identification of two regions in the amino-terminal domain of ActA involved in the actin comet tail formation by *Listeria monocytogenes*. *EMBO J* 1997; 16: 1531-40.
35. Niebuhr K, Ebel F, Frank R, Reinhard M, Domann E, Carl UD, Walter U, Gertler FB, Wehland J, Chakraborty T. A novel proline-rich motif present in ActA of *Listeria monocytogenes* and cytoskeletal proteins is the ligand for the EVH1 domain, a protein module present in the Ena/VASP family. *EMBO J* 1997; 16: 5433-44.

36. Mourrain P, Lasa I, Gautreau A, Gouin E, Pugsley A, Cossart P. ActA is a dimer. *Proc Natl Acad Sci USA* 1997; 94: 10034-9.
37. Finlay BB, Falkow S. Common themes in microbial pathogenicity. II. *Microbiol Mol Biol Rev* 1997; 61: 136-69.
38. Dramsi S, Cossart P. Intracellular pathogens and the actin cytoskeleton. *Ann Rev Cell Dev Biol* 1998 (in press).

Bacterial toxins in the gastrointestinal tract

Recent advances in the pathogenesis of gastrointestinal bacterial infections.
P. Rampal, P. Boquet, eds. John Libbey Eurotext, Paris © 1998, pp. 127-134.

Enterotoxigenic *Escherichia coli*

Patrice Boquet

INSERM U 452, Faculté de Médecine de Nice, 28, avenue de Valombrose, 06107 Nice Cedex 2, France

Enterotoxigenic *Escherichia coli* (ETEC) are among the most important causes of diarrhea. ETEC may produce 4 types of toxin: the heat-stable (Sta and STb) the heat labile (LT1 and LT2) enterotoxins, the cytolethal distending toxin (CDT) and the cytotoxic necrotizing factors (CNF1 and CNF2).
STa is associated with disease in both human and animals, and STb is found mostly associated with diarrhea in piglets. LT1 is associated in both humans and animals and LT2 has been found in animals. CDT has been isolated from *E. coli* of a small number of children with diarrhea on the fact that this toxin produced elongation of CHO cells followed by progressive cellular distension and cytotoxicity. CNF1 and CNF2, which produce massive reorganization of the actin cytoskeleton on HEp-2 cells, have been associated mostly with extraintestinal infections (eg septicemia and urinary tract infection) but also in enteritis in humans and animals. Since the molecular mechanism of CNF1 has been recently demonstrated, we shall begin this short review on CNF. An exhaustive review on enteric bacterial toxins may be consulted for certain details [1].

E. coli cytotoxic necrotizing factors (CNF1 and CNF2)

CNF1, discovered by Caprioli and colleagues, as a cell-associated product of *E. coli* strains isolated from young children with diarrhea, causes necrosis of rabbit skin and multinucleation of different types of tissue culture cells [2]. A second type of CNF (CNF2) was then found in extracts of certain *E. coli* strains isolated from calves with enteritis [3]. CNF2 and CNF1 are immunologically related and similar in apparent molecular weight (110-115 kDa). CNF1 is chromosomally encoded in a 620 Kb pathogenicity island (PAI II) containing the α-hemolysin and a fimbriae gene (PRS) [4] but also many others *orf*. Some of these *orf* have sequence similarities with known enterobacteria virulence factors. CNF2 gene is located on a large transmissible F-like plasmid (Vir).

CNF1 and CNF2 are encoded by a single structural gene with a low GC content (35%) [5, 6]. This finding suggests a relatively recent acquisition of the *cnf* gene by *E. coli* whose overall GC content is around 50%. Analysis of the deduced amino acid sequences of CNF1 and CNF2 showed that the two toxins are quite similar (85% identical and 99% conserved residues over 1,014 amino acids). Additionally, CNFs are predicted to be relatively hydrophilic proteins with two putative hydrophobic transmembrane domains partially overlapped by two predicted α helices. No classical signal peptide sequence was found in CNFs N-terminal 50 residues. CNFs share regions of homologous amino acids with two other bacterial toxins: *Pasteurella multocida* toxin (PMT) and the dermonecrotic toxin of *Bordetella pertussis* (DNT). CNFs, PMT and DNT form the new family of dermonecrotic toxins [7].

CNF1 is able to provoke a remarkable reorganization of F-actin structures in cultured cells [8]. This toxin induces intense formation of stress fibers, focal contacts, membrane folding and retraction fibers. Reorganization of the F-actin cytoskeleton by CNF1 results in the cells unability to undergo cytokinesis. Cells treatment for over 24 h with CNF1, at concentrations as low as 10 pg/ml, gives rise to extremely flat large multinucleated cells containing numerous stress fibers.

Treatment of HEp-2 cells with CNF1, for increasing lengths of time (from 4 to 72 h), induces an augmented ability of the cells to ingest latex beads [9]. Macropinocytosis is totally blocked when CNF1 treated cells are incubated with the F-actin disrupting drug cytochalasin B demonstrating clearly that the process is F-actin dependent [9]. In addition, non-invasive bacteria such as *Listeria innocua* are found to be as invasive as *L. monocytogenes* when incubated with HEp-2 cells pretreated with CNF1 [9]. Only *L. innocua* harboring a plasmid containing the listeriolysin gene were found to multiply in the cytoplasm of HEp-2 cells treated with CNF1, indicating that macropinocytosis of bacteria was associated with formation of vacuoles [9].

Incubation of intestinal T84, cells cultivated polarized on filters, with CNF1 does not influence transepithelial resistance suggesting that barrier function and surface polarity are not affected by the toxin. Incubation of T84 cells with CNF1 induced F-actin accumulation, impaired PMNs transepithelial migration (in either the luminal-to-basolateral or the basolateral-to luminal directions). Thus CNF1-activated Rho, by reorganizing F-actin structures in intestinal epithelial cells, induces a decrease ability of PMNs to cross the epithelial barrier. Furthermore, CNF1 effaces intestinal cells microvilli allowing a better bacterial adherence and probably also an improved growth of microbes by impairing absorbtion of nutrients by microvilli [10].

In serum starved Swiss 3T3 cells growth factors such as EGF, PDGF bombesin and certain lipids such as lysophosphatidic acid (LPA) can stimulate the reorganization of F-actin structures, through small p21 Ras-like GTP-binding proteins of the Rho family [11]. Stimulation *via* Rac was shown to induce ruffling. Formation of stress fibers and focal contacts was observed upon the stimulation of the Rho GTPase. Finally activation of Cdc42 was shown to induce formation of filopodia. Rho regulates the actin cytoskeleton through two main mechanisms: 1/ bundling and contractility of actin filaments by inhibition, *via* phosporylation by the Rho kinase, of the myosin light chain phosphatase (MLCP) 2/ actin polymerization by formation of PIP2 through activation of the Ptds-5P kinase. PIP2 is though to induce actin polymerization by uncapping barbed end actin filaments [12].

CNF1 induces cells actin reorganization by stimulating permanently the Rho protein. The first hint for this activity was shown as follows: when the cytosol from HEp-2 cells previously incubated with CNF1 was ADP-ribosylated with exoenzyme C3 it was observed that the Rho protein had a molecular weight shifted to a slightly higher value. This result indicated a possible post-translational modification of the GTP-binding protein in CNF1 treated cells [6]. CNF1-induced electrophoretic shift of Rho is not due to a block in prenylation (post translational modification of the carboxy-terminus ends of small GTP-binding proteins) nor to a phosphorylation of Rho [6]. CNF1 was shown then to modify directly *in vitro* Rho without the need of cellular co-factors [13]. Microsequencing of CNF1-modified Rho showed that there was a single modification in the CNF1-treated GTPase compared to wild type. Rho glutamine 63 was changed into a glutamic acid [13]. Therefore, CNF1 exerts a specific deamidase activity. An identical activity for CNF1 on Rho has been reported using mass spectrometry [14]. Specific deamidation is a hitherto undescribed activity for a bacterial toxin. Indeed, toxin enzymatic activities described at the present time are ADP-ribosylation, depurination, metallo-protease, glucosyl transferase and adenylate cycling.

CNF1 has a deamidase catalytic activity on Rho glutamine 63. The equivalent amino acid of Rho glutamine 63 in p21 Ras is glutamine 61. Rho glutamine 63 is known to be an important residue for the intrinsic and RhoGAP mediated GTPase of Rho [15]. Both CNF1-treated Rho and mutated Rho on glutamine 63 into glutamic acid (RhoQ63E exhibit a mobility shift, upon electrophoresis, identical to CNF1-treated Rho). CNF1-treated Rho and RhoQ63E nucleotide dissociation rate was increased by 2 orders of magnitude but the RhoGAP activity was totally impaired on both CNF1-treated Rho and RhoQ63E. Thus, CNF1 allows Rho to be permanently bound with GTP enhancing the activity on Rho on Rho effectors. CNF1 deamidase activity is borne by the 30kDa carboxy-terminus end of the molecule [6]. On the other hand, the cell binding moiety of CNF1 is localized in the amino-terminus of the molecule [6]. CNF1 has thus a toxin architecture comparable to *Pseudomonas aeruginosa* exotoxin A [16]. Comparisons of sequence homologies between the different dermonecrotic toxins CNF1, CNF2, DNT and PMT has revealed that CNF1 and CNF2 are highly homologous, sharing both comparable domains for enzymatic and cell binding domains. DNT, however, is a toxin which has a high homologies with CNFs for the catalytic domain but differs strongly with CNFs at the level of the cell binding domain. PMT on the other hand, differs strongly with CNFs and DNT at the level of its putative catalytic domain but has a strong homology with cell binding domains of CNFs [6].

Heat stable enterotoxins (ST)

This family of enterotoxins encompasses 2 main members: STa and STb. STa is a cystein-rich peptide of 18 amino-acids (aa). The toxin is encoded by the transposon-associated *esta* gene located on a plasmid [17] STa is produced under the form of a 72 aa precursor cleaved by the signal peptidase type 1 to a 53 aa polypeptide. The 53 aa STa precursor is translocated to the periplasm where three intramolecular disulfide bounds, absolutly required for the toxin activity, are catalyzed by the DsbA protein prior to secretion by *E. coli*. Extracellularly, a second proteolytic event occurs which cleaves the STa into a 18 amino acids polypeptide (mature form of STa). Residues 11 to 14 of mature STa (Asn-Pro-Ala-Cys) are strictly conserved in all members of the ST toxin family and partially conserved in the endogenous hormone guanylin [18]. STa residues 5 to 17 confer full binding to its receptor and enterotoxic activities. STa binds to a receptor localized in the intestinal brush border membrane. This receptor, the guanylate cyclase (GC) (a 120 kDa MW protein) is embeded in the membrane and is present in all the digestive tract although in decreasing number from the small intestine to the rectum. GC is present in large amount in young children and decrease rapidly with increasing age [19]. This may explain why diarrhea induced by STa are more severe in young children than in adults. After STa binding GC is activated. The mechanism of this activation appears to be the result of a change of GC conformation inhibiting the kinase domain activity of GC since genetic deletion of the kinase domain provokes the permanent activation of GC and its unresponsiveness to STa.

Activation of GC by STa increases the level of intracellular cyclic GMP that stimulates chloride secretion resulting in the inhibition of NaC1 absorbtion. Activation of chloride secretion may occur *via* activation of a cGMP-dependent kinase present in the apical membrane of enterocytes which ultimatly activates the chloride channel CFTR. However, this is still unclear. It has been reported that the secretory response to STa in T84 cells involved F-actin reargments only at the basal pole of these cells [20].

STb a 71 amino acids is plasmid encoded (estB) [21]. STb is processed in the periplasmic space into a 48 amino acids polypeptide containing 4 cysteines forming 2 disulfide bonds. STb is not processed further in the extracellular medium. The receptor for STb is still unknown. STb does not activate the guanylate cyclase. STb does not appear to have an effect on human small intestine consistent with the infrequent occurrence in human disease of *E. coli* strains expressing STb. In mouse intestine STb induces histologic changes consisting in a loss of villus epithelial cells. No secretion of chloride has been found. It seems that STb, by acting *via* a pertussis toxin sensitive heterotrimeric G-protein, stimulates a dose dependent increase in intracellular calcium.

E. coli heat-labile enterotoxins LT

LT1 and LT2 enterotoxin are closely related to cholera toxin (CT). LT1 shares 80% sequence identity with the A and B subunits of CT. On the other hand LT2 shares only 55% identity with the A subunit of CT but essentially no homology with the B subunit of CT [22]. LT1 shares many similarities with CT in term of receptor binding and enzymatic activity. However, *E. coli* strains producing LT1 produce mild diseases compared to CT. LT1, as CT, is an A-B subunit toxin (A/B ratio, 1:5) where B is the subunit (11.6 kDa) which binds to its GM1 ganglioside receptor and A is an enzymatic intracellular acting component. The A subunit consists of two components generated by proteolysis. The A1 (21.8 kDa) is an ADP-ribosyltransferase and A2 (5.4 kDa) links A1 to the B subunits. X-ray crystallography shows that the structure of LT1 consists of 5 B subunits forming a pentamer with a central pore, where the carboxy terminus of A2 is located. A2 is linked, by an alpha helix, to the A1 subunit [23]. The A1 subunit ADP-ribosylates the Gs alpha chain of an heterotrimeric GTP-binding protein which controls the activity of adenylate cyclase (Gs). ADP-ribosylation of alpha Gs by LT1/CT occurs only in the presence of the small GTP-binding protein ARF leading to the inhibition of the GTPase activity of alpha Gs [24]. This result in an intracellular activation of adenylate cyclase thus to elevation of cyclic AMP. LT I, as CT, enters cells by endocytosis, is transferred to early endosomes then to late endosomes where apparently there is a separation between the A1 and the A2/B5 subunits [25]. The A1 subunit alone is transferred from late endosomes to the trans-Golgi network whereas the A2/B5 fragment, following transfer to lysosomes is degraded [25]. The A1 LT1 subunit is transported in a retrograde fashion to the endoplasmic reticulum where apparently it enters into the cytosol [25]. That way the enzymatic moiety of LT1 is delivered directly at the cell baso-lateral pole where Gs alpha subunits sit.

Elevation of cAMP by LT1 results in a slow onset of inhibition of NaC1 absorbtion and stimulation of Cl^- secretion similar (except in time course) to the effect of STa. LT1 most probably, by elevating cAMP, activates a kinase cAMP dependent (A-kinase) which up-regulates chloride secretion, by phosphorylation of the CFTR channel. However, LT1 activity on intestinal cells may induce others effects. Prostaglandins of the E series (PGE1 and PGE2) and PAF (platelet activating factor) are also implicated in CT/LT1 activities [26, 27]. LT1 by increasing cAMP increase production of PAF. which in turn, stimulates production of PGE2.

LTI like CT may also alters the activity of the enteric nervous system. Serotonin (5-HT) and VIP are released into the lumen small bowel *in vivo* after treatment with CT [28]. There are some evidence that CT (thus probably LT1) can binds and activates VIP-containing neurons in the intestinal sub-mucosa of guinea pigs [29].

LT 2, which shares many similarities in term of structure and activities with CT/LT1, has been isolated essentially from animals. LT2 subunit B, does not bind to GM1 gangliosides. LT2 is in fact divided into two subgroups: LT2a and LT2b on the basis of their amino acids sequences. LT2a binds best GD1b gangliosides and LT2b GD1a gangliosides.

E. coli cytolethal distending toxin (CDT)

Cytolethal distending toxins belong to an emerging toxin family whose members have been found in several unrelated bacterial species including: *E. coli*, *Shigella dysenteriae*, *Campylobacter* sp. and *Haemophylus ducrey*. The genetic structure coding for CDT is made in all cases by three adjacent or slightly overlapping chromosomal genes (cdtA, cdtB and cdtC) [30] which encode three subunits of A (27 kDa), B (29 kDa) and C (20 kDa). The biological activity of CDT on cultured cells consists in the induction of giant elongated cells (in CHO cells) and an inhibition of cell division at the G2/M stage of the cell cycle. This mitotic block induces cell death after 3 to 5 days of toxin activity. A recent study indicates that cells treated by CDT, accumulate in late G2 due to the absence of cdc2 dephosphorylation [31]. According to this study CDT might interfere with a cell transduction cascade, initiated in the S phase (during DNA replication), called DNA damage checkpoint which is the mechanism that detects damaged DNA. However the nature of the CDT subunit inducing this effect and its exact molecular intracellular activity is still unknown.

References

1. Sears CL, Kaper JB. Enteric bacterial toxins: mechanisms of action and linkage to intestinal secretion. *Microbiol Rev* 1996; 60: 167-215.
2. Caprioli A, Falbo V, Roda LG, Ruggeri FM, Zona C. Partial purification and characterization of an *Escherichia coli* toxic factor that induces morphological cell alterations. *Infect Immun* 1983; 39: 1300-6.
3. De Rycke J, Gonzales EA, Blanco J, Oswald E, Blanco M, Boivin R. Evidence for two types of cytotoxic necrotizing factor in human and clinical isolates. *J Clin Microbiol* 1990; 28: 694-9.
4. Blum G, Falbo V, Caprioli A, Hacker J. Gene cluster encoding the cytotoxic necrotizing factor type 1 Prs fimbriae and α hemolysin from the pathogenicity island II of the uropathogenic *Escherichia coli* stain 96. *FEMS Microbiol Lett* 1995; 126: 189-96.
5. Falbo V, Pace T, Picci L, Pizzi E, Caprioli A. Isolation and nucleotide sequence of the gene encoding cytotoxic necrotizing factor type I. *Infect Immun* 1993; 61: 4909-14.
6. Oswald E, Sugai M, Labigne A, Wu HC, Fiorentini C, Boquet P, O'Brien A. Cytotoxic necrotizing factor type 2 produced by virulent *Escherichia coli* modifies the small GTP-binding protein Rho involved in assembly of actin stress fibers. *Proc Natl Acad Sci USA* 1994; 91: 3814-8.
7. Lemichez E, Flatau G, Bruzzone M, Boquet P, Gauthier M. Molecular localization of the *Escherichia coli* cytotoxic necrotizing factor CNF1 cell-binding and catalytic domains. *Mol Microbiol* 1997; 24: 1061-70.
8. Fiorentini C, Arancia G, Caprioli A, Falbo V, Ruggeri FM, Donelli G. Cytoskeletal changes induced in HEp-2 cells by the cytotoxic necrotizing factor of *Escherichia coli*. *Toxicon* 1988; 26: 1047-56.
9. Falzano L, Fiorentini C, Donelli G, Michel E, Kocks C, Cossart P, Cabanié L, Oswald E, Boquet P. Induction of phagocytic behaviour in human epithelial cells by *Escherichia coli* cytotoxic necrotizing factor type I. *Mol Microbiol* 1993; 9: 1247-54.

10. Hofman P, Flatau G, Selva E, Gauthier M, Piche M, Fiorentini C, Rossi B, Boquet P. *Escherichia coli* cytotoxic necrotizing factor I (CNF1) effaces microvilli and decreases transmigration of polymorphonuclear leukocytes in intestinal T84 epithelial cell monolayers. *Infect Immun* 1998; under press.
11. Tapon N, Hall A. Rho, Rac and Cdc42 GTPases regulate the organization of the actin cytoskeleton. *Curr Opin Cell Biol* 1997; 9: 86-92.
12. Hall A. Rho GTPases and the actin cytoskeleton. *Science* 1998; 279: 509-14.
13. Flatau G, Lemichez E, Gauthier M, Chardin P, Paris S, Fiorentini C, Boquet P. Toxin-induced activation of the G-protein Rho by deamidation of glutamine. *Nature* 1997; 387: 729-33.
14. Schmidt G, Sehr P, Wilm M, Selzer J, Mann M, Aktories K. Gln 63 of Rho is deamidated by *Escherichia coli* cytotoxic necrotizing factor 1. *Nature* 1997; 387: 725-8.
15. Rittinger K, Walker P A, Eccleston JF, Smerdon SJ, Gamblin SJ. Structure at 1.65 Angstrom of RhoA and its GTPase-activating protein in complex with transition state analog. *Nature* 1997; 389: 758-62.
16. Allured VS, Collier RJ, Carroll SF, McKay DB. Structure of exotoxin A of *Pseudomonas aeruginosa* at 3.0 Angstrom resolution. *Proc Natl Acad Sci USA* 1986; 83: 1320-4.
17. So M, Mc Carthy BJ. Nucleotide sequence of the bacterial transposon Tn 1681 encoding heat-stable (ST) toxin and its identification in enteropathogenic *Escherichia coli* strains. *Proc Natl Acad Sci USA* 1980; 77: 4011-5.
18. Kuhn M, Aderman K, Jähne J, Forssmann WG, Rechkemmer G. Segmental difference in the effects of guanylin and *Escherichia coli* heat-stable enterotoxin on Cl^- secretion in human gut. *J Physiol (London)* 1994; 479: 433-40.
19. Cohen NB, Guarino A, Shulka R, Giannella RA. Age-related differences in receptors for *Escherichia coli* heat-stable enterotoxin in the small and large intestine of children. *Gastroenterology* 1988; 94: 367-73.
20. Matthews JB, Smith JA, Tally KJ, Awtrey CS, Nguyen H, Rich J, Madara JL. Na^+ K^+ 2 Cl^- cotransport and Cl^- secretion evoked by heat-stable enterotoxin is microfilament dependent in T84 cells. *Am J Physiol* 1994; 265: G373-G378.
21. Piken RM, Mazaitis AJ, Maas WK, Rey M, Heyneiker H. Nucleotide sequence of the gene for heat-stable enterotoxin 2 of *Escherichia coli*. *Infect Immun* 1983; 42: 269-75.
22. Pickett CL, Twiddy EM, Coker C, Holmes RA, Cloning, nucleotide sequence and hybridization studies of the type 2b heat-labile enterotoxin gene of *Escherichia coli*. *J Bact* 1989; 171: 4945-52.
23. Sixma TK, Pronk SE, Kalk KM, Wartna ES, Van Zanten BA, Witholt B, Hol WG. Crystal structure of a cholera toxin-related heat-labile enterotoxin from *E. coli*. *Nature* 1991; 351: 371-7.
24. Moss J, Vaughan M. Activation of cholera toxin and heat-labile enterotoxins by ADP-ribosylation factors, a family of 20 kDa guanine nucleotide binding proteins. *Mol Microbiol* 1991; 5: 2621-7.
25. Majoul IV, Bastiaens PIH, Soling HM. Transport of an external lys-Asp-Glu-Leu (KDEL) protein from the plasma membrane to the endoplasmic reticulum: studies with cholera toxin in Vero cells. *J Cell Biol* 1996; 133: 777-89.
26. Peterson JW, Ochoa LG. Role of prostaglandins and cAMP in the secretory effects of cholera toxin. *Science* 1989; 245: 857-9.
27. Guerrant RL, Fang GD, Thielman MH, Fonteles MC. Role of platelet activating factor (PAF) in the intestinal epithelial secretory and chinese hamster ovary (CHO) cell cytoskeletal responses to cholera toxin. *Proc Natl Acad Sci USA* 1994; 91: 9655-8.
28. Nilsson O, Cassuto J, Larsson PA, Jodal M, Lindberg P, Ahlman H, Dahlström A, Lundgren O. 5-hydroxy tryptamine and cholera secretion: a histochemical and physiological study in cats. *Gut* 1983; 24: 542-8.

29. Jiang MA, Kirchgessner A, Gershon MD, Surprenant A. Cholera toxin-sensitive neuron in guinea-pig submucosal plexus. *Am J Physiol* 1993; 264: G86-G94.
30. Scott DA, Kaper JB. Cloning and sequencing of the genes encoding *Escherichia coli* cytolethal distending toxin. *Infect Immun* 1994; 62: 244-51.
31. Comayras C, Tasca C, Péres SY, Ducommun B, Oswald E, de Rycke J. *Escherichia coli* cytolethal distending toxin blocks the HeLa cell cycle at the G2/M transistion by preventing cdc2 protein kinase dephosphorylation and activation. *Infect Immun* 1997; 65: 5088-95.

Recent advances in the pathogenesis of gastrointestinal bacterial infections.
P. Rampal, P. Boquet, eds. John Libbey Eurotext, Paris © 1998, pp. 135-142.

Clostridium difficile

Ingo Just

Institut für Pharmakologie und Toxikologie der Albert-Ludwigs-Universität Freiburg, Hermann-Herder-Str. 5, D-79104 Freiburg, Germany

Clostridium difficile, a Gram-positive anaerobic bacterium, is the causative agent of the antibiotic-associated pseudomembranous colitis (PMC). *C. difficile* is involved in almost all cases of PMC and in about 25% of cases of antibiotic-associated diarrhoea. About 50% of newborn infants are carrier of *C. difficile* without symptoms whereas only 1% of the adults are asymptomatic carriers.
C. difficile-caused diarrhoea is triggered by therapy with broad-spectrum antibiotics which have activity against enterobacteria. The physiological colonic flora suppresses the growth of *C. difficile* through an unknown mechanism. Antibiotics decrease and disturb the normal flora thereby creating conditions which allow *C. difficile* to colonise and grow. In the vegetative form *C. difficile* produces toxin A and toxin B which are the two major pathogenicity factors. Clindamycin was the first antibiotic to be identified as inducer of the PMC. Today, broadspectrum penicillins and cephalosporins produce most frequently the PMC, not because of the high incidence of this side effect but because of their wide spread use. *C. difficile* infection affects mainly elder people and hospitalysed patients. One obvious reason is the widely and increasingly use of antibiotics. However in hospitals, the nosocomial infection is important due to contamination of wards with *C. difficile* spores [1].
The clinical symptoms vary from mild diarrhoea to pseudomembranous colitis. Often *C. difficile* infection causes a sudden onset of a mild to moderate diarrhoea, accompanied by spasmodic abdominal pain but without general symptoms. The symptoms normally begin during or shortly after antibiotic therapy and subside spontanously after cessation of therapy. Patients with severe colitis but without formation of pseudomembranes have profuse abdominal pain and distension accompanied by nausea, fever and dehydration. The symptoms of the pseudomembranous colitis are in general more marked. Sigmoidoscopy or coloscopy reveal the characteristic yellowish plaques which are in diameter up to 1 cm. These plaques are distributed in a patchy manner, the intervening mucosa is normal or mildly erythematous. The histological feature of the PMC is characterised by patchy epithelial

necrosis up to epithelial ulceration. The so-called "pseudomembranes" which are composed of mucus, fibrin, leukocytes, and cellular debris, are located in the focus of the ulceration. The most severe form of the PMC is the life-threatening fulminant colitis which has the symptoms of an acute abdomen [2].

The laboratory diagnosis is based on the detection of the *C. difficile* toxins in stool samples. The most rapid tests are commercial enzyme linked immunoassy kits (ELISA) which rely on the detection of toxin A or toxin A and B. To increase sensitivity and specificity, *C. difficile* can be cultured and then subcultured followed by an ELISA to detect toxin-producing *C. difficile* strains.

The first step of the treatment of the *C. difficile*-induced diarrhoea/colitis is the discontinuation of the antibiotic therapy if there is no vital indication. The mild to moderate forms cease spontaneously after discontinuation of the antibiotic therapy. The more severe forms need antibiotic therapy to eradicate *C. difficile.* Metronidazole or vancomycin given orally are the drugs of choice, which are usually administered for about ten days. Both drugs are equally potent to resolve the colitis by about 95%. Severe and debilitating diarrhoea needs, in addition, the preservation of the fluid and electrolyte balance. Relapses are not uncommon (10 to 20% of the patients) and metronidazole or vancomycin therapy frequently fails to prevent relapses. One alternative is the treatment with the yeast *Saccharomyces boullardii* which is reported to reduce the failure rate (reviews [2-6]).

There are many factors by which pathogenic strains of *C. difficile* mediate diarrhoea and colitis, comprising the presence of fimbriae, proteases and toxins [7]. The most important and best studied are two toxins, designated enterotoxin (toxin A) and cytotoxin (toxin B). *C. difficile* strains which do not produce toxins are not pathogenic. Both toxins are exotoxins which are single-chain polypeptides having molecular weights of 308 kDa (toxin A) and 270 kDA (toxin B), respectively.

In animal models (explanted duodenum of rabbits), the enterotoxin (toxin A) causes inflammatory responses, fluid accumulation and necrosis in the gut. In this *in vivo* model toxin B alone is inactive as enterotoxin but the combination with subthreshhold concentrations of toxin A elicits some enterotoxic effects. In cultured cell lines, toxin B is a potent cytoxin whereas toxin A is about one hundred to thousand fold less cytotoxic. However, recent studies demonstrated that toxin B is more potent or at least comparable potent on human colonic mucosa and human colonic cancer T84 cells than toxin A to cause morphological damage and decrease in transepithelial resistance. After parental application, however, both toxins are lethal at comparable concentrations [3, 8].

In cultured cells, both toxins induce the same morphological changes, however, with different potency. The most prominent effect is the depolymerisation of the actin cytoskeleton. Initially, the stress fibres disappear, followed by shrinking whereby retraction fibres remain at the beginning of the intoxication. Eventually, the cells are completely rounded having a significantly reduced cell volume [9]. Because the toxins exhibit their cytotoxic activity at very low concentrations (femtomolar range) it was clear from the beginning that the mode of action must be enzymic. In fact, toxin A and toxin B have been shown to mono-glucosylate the low molecular GTP-binding proteins of the Rho family. Using UDP-glucose as cosubstrate, the toxins transfer the glucose moiety to a threonine residue. The O-glycosidic bound glucose renders the GTP-binding proteins inactive thereby inhibiting downstream signalling.

This type of modification is a novel cytotoxic mechanism by which bacteria act on eukaryotic cells [10, 11].
The Rho proteins belong to the Ras superfamily of low molecular mass GTP-binding proteins (GTPases) which are involved in the intracellular signal transduction to serve as molecular switches. These GTPases are characterised by their molecular weight (18-28 kDa), their C-terminal polyisoprenylation and their property to bind and hydrolyse guanine nucleotides. They are inactive in the GDP-bound state and binding of GTP induces activation resulting in downstream signalling. The transition between inactive and active state is controlled by several regulatory proteins: The guanine nucleotide exchange factors (GEF) promote the exchange of nucleotides and binding of GTP; the GTPase-activating proteins (GAP) strongly stimulates the low intrinsic GTPase activity to terminate the activated state; the guanine nucleotide dissociation inhibitor (GDI) traps the inactive GDP-bound form in a high affinity complex. Binding of GTP induces changes in the conformation which allows binding to the so-called effector protein. Effectors are often serine/threonine kinases which possess a Rho-binding domain. Binding of Rho results in activation of the kinase (*e.g.* ROKα/Rho kinase) which phosphorylates downstream targets. In addition to kinases, Rho effectors comprise also multidomain proteins without enzymic activity (rhotekin, rhophilin) which may serve as nucleus for multimolecular complexes to connect different signalling pathways *(figure 1)*.

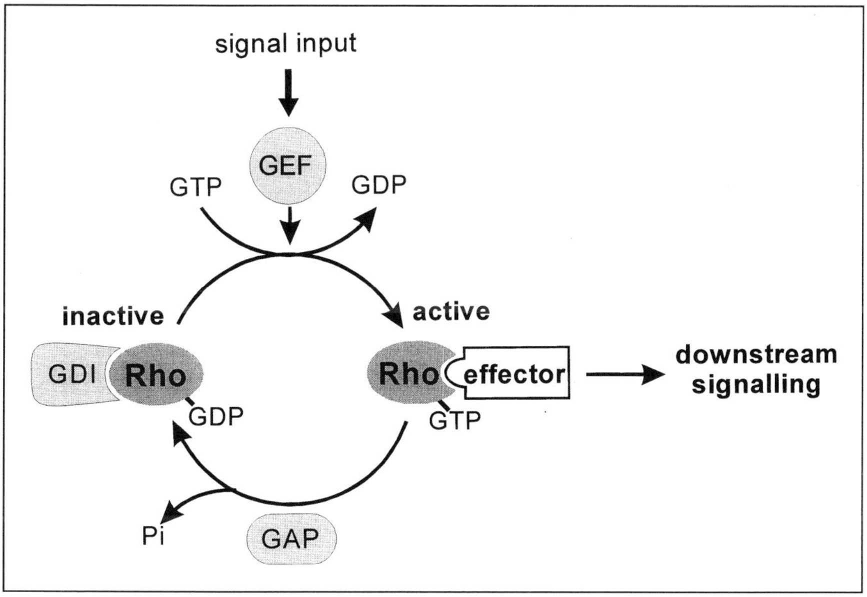

Figure 1. Signalling cycle of the Rho proteins.

The best characterised members of the Rho subfamily are Rho, Rac and Cdc42. In general, they are involved in the regulation of the dynamic actin cytoskeleton. Each of them, however, regulates distinct structures: Rho governs the formation of stress fibres and focal adhesions, Rac is involved in membrane ruffling and Cdc42 in the formation of filopodia. The best understood functional modul is the formation of the stress fibres: Rac and Rho regulates the phosphatidyl-inositide (4)-phosphate-5-kinase (PI-5-kinase) to form PIP_2. PIP_2 stimulates actin polymerisation and filament growth through interaction with several actin-binding proteins (*e.g.* gelsolin, profilin). The stress fibres, a supra organisation of actin filaments, are govern by the RhoA-dependent Rho-Kinase which phosphorylates the myosin light chain thereby activating the actin-myosin system in non-muscle cells. The membrane attachment of the stress fibres is managed through the ERM proteins (ezrin, radixin, moesin). These bifunctional proteins bind through their N-terminal part to transmembrane proteins (CD44 or ICAM proteins) and interact through their C-terminal part with the actin filaments. This interaction is essential for Rho-governed cytoskeletal changes.

The family of Rho protein are involved in several cellular events. The *table I* gives only a short overview of the multiple functions reported on the Rho proteins:

Table I. Overview of the multiple functions reported on the Rho proteins

General involvement in detailed function	
Organisation of the actin cytoskeleton	Stress fibres, membrane ruffling, filopodia formation, cell adhesion, cell-cell contact, cell morphology, cell motility
Membrane trafficking	Endocytosis, exocytosis, phagocytosis
Smooth muscle contraction	Calcium sensitisation
Phospholipid metabolism	PI-5-kinase, PLD, PLC
Cell cycle progression	Transition from G1 to S phase
Reactive oxygen species (ROS)	NADPH oxidase of neutrophils
Transcriptional activation	JNK, p38RK, NFκB
Cell transformation	
Apoptosis	

Rho/Rac/Cdc42-dependent signal pathways are stimulated by receptor-thyrosine kinases (PDGF for Rac) and by G-protein-coupled receptors (LPA for Rho, bradykinin for Cdc42). The regulation of the exchange factors (GEFs) which directly promote activation of the Rho proteins is quite unclear but there are some data that thyrosine phosphorylation or phospholipid (PIP_2) binding is involved. The functional hierarchy of Rho proteins (Cdc42 activates Rac and Rac activates Rho) and the crosstalk between the protooncogene Ras and Rac is also part of the upstream regulation of the Rho proteins. (Reviews on the Rho proteins [12-17].)

Functional consequences of glucosylation of Rho proteins: The acceptor amino acid of glucosylation (threonine-37) is located in the effector domain (amino acids 30-42). Through this domain the low molecular G-proteins couple to the downstream effector proteins which result in downstream signalling. The hydroxyl group of threonine-37 is involved in the binding of the β- and γ-phosphate of GTP through coordination of the Mg^{2+} ion. A glucose moiety attached to this residue causes alteration of Rho functions [18, 19]:

- Activation by exchange factors (GEFs) is reduced but not completely inhibited.
- Coupling to the effector proteins is completely blocked.
- Intrinsic GTPase is reduced but GAP-stimulated GTPase is completely inhibited.

Thus, the crucial step of downstream signalling, the effector coupling, is completely inhibited. Thus, glucosylation switches off the function of the Rho proteins and all Rho-dependent signal pathways are blocked, *i.e.*, depolymerisation of the actin cytoskeleton, inhibition of cell motility, superoxide anion production by neutrophils, etc.

Structure of the toxins. Toxin A and toxin B, which are coproduced by the clostridia, are single-chain polypetides with molecular masses of 308 kDa and 270 kDa, respectively. Both toxins are cloned and sequenced revealing an amino acid sequence homology of 63% and an identical structural composition [20]. The polypeptides are composed of three functional domains: i) the N-terminal catalytic domain, ii) the intermediate translocation domain, and iii) the C-terminal receptor binding domain [21-23] *(figure 2).*

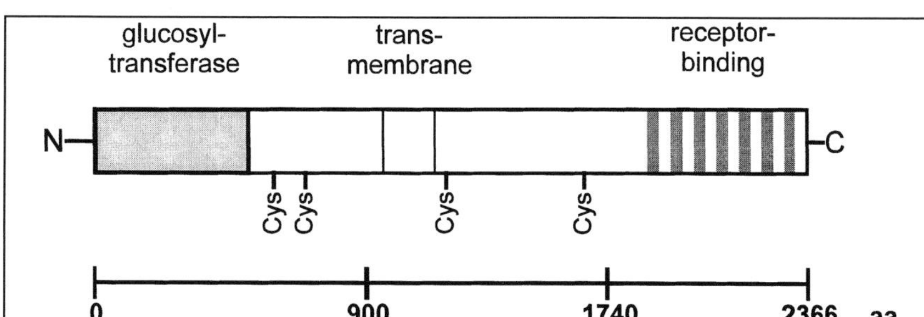

Figure 2. Structure of toxin B.

By expression of the separate fragments of toxin B, it has been demonstrated that the N-terminal part (residues 1-546 from 2,366 residues in total) harbours the mono-glucosyltransferase activity [24]. Neither the conserved cysteine residues (Cys-595 and Cys-698) nor the putative nucleotide binding domain (located within these two cysteines) are essential for the enzymic activity. The toxins cleave the cosubstrate UDP-glucose and transfer the glucose group to the acceptor amino acid threonine to form an O-glycosidic linkage. Comparable to eukaryotic glucosyltransferases, the *C. difficile* toxins need Mn^{2+} ions for their catalytic activity. Microinjection of the cell impermeable N-terminal fragment induces the same cytoskeletal effects as the holotoxin applied to the intact cells. Thus, the cytotoxic effects of toxin B are very likely caused by their mono-glucosyltransferase activity.

The intermediate part contains a helical transmembrane domain which is very likely to serve as the translocation domain. This domain is believed to translocate the toxin or a part of it from an acidic endosomal compartment to the cytosol where the toxin can meet and modify the Rho proteins.

The C-terminal part, covering a third of the molecule, consists of series of repeat units which show homology to the carbohydrate binding domain of streptococcal glucosyltransferases [25]. The monoclonal antibody PCG-4 used in most diagnostic kits recognises epitopes of this toxin part. It has been shown that toxin A binds to the terminal carbohydrate structure Galα1-3Galβ1-4GlcNAc which is possibly part of the glycoprotein receptor of toxin A. More recently, the membranous sucrase-isomaltase glycoprotein was identified as toxin A receptor in rabbit ileal brush border [26]. However, this receptor seems not to be of general importance, because it is not expressed in many toxin-sensitive tissues (*e.g.* human colon). The nature of the toxin B receptor is still unclear but it is clear that toxin A and toxin B receptors are different. The repetitive structure of the receptor domains of toxin A as well as toxin B argues for a modular organisation of this domain. By this modular structure, the toxin can bind to several possibly identical receptors to induce clustering followed by endocytosis. The current concept of toxin A/B entry into the cells is that the toxins bind to their cellular receptor *via* a lectin-like binding. The toxins are taken up by a receptor-mediated endocytosis followed by translocation from an acidic endosomal compartment to the cytosol where the toxins or fragments of them exhibit mono-glucosyltransferase activity to modify Rho proteins [22, 27-29].

In animal models it has been shown that toxin A induces fluid secretion, inflammation and histological damage. These outcomes are mediated by direct effects of the toxin on the intestinal epithelial cell layer to open tight junctions resulting in increased permeability. Toxin B, which is non-toxic when applied alone in these models, gains access to subepithelial compartments to exhibit effects. The toxins are reported to be involved in the release of mediators as leukotriens, prostaglandines, PAF and histamine which themselves are modulators of the intestinal permeability. Furthermore, the recruitment of neutrophils is caused by interleukins (IL-1 and IL-8); this toxin A effect is blocked by pertussis toxin indicating the involvement of a G-protein coupled signal pathway [30, 31]. (Review [4, 8].)

These data of direct and indirect effects of toxin A effects on intestinal cells are contradictory to the finding of the intracellular mode of action through glucosylation of the low molecular mass GTP binding Rho proteins. As can be deduced from Rho signalling pathways, *e.g.* inactivation of Rho should block neutrophil activation and cytokine release as well mast cell degranulation.

To reconcile both concepts, two different mode of actions are to be postulated: I. A membrane receptor effect of the toxins by which more or less immediately the signal is transmitted by coupled G-proteins to the intracellular space. II. An intracellular effect appearing after cell entry of the toxins and exhibiting their enzymic activity. However, the action of the toxins through membrane receptor(s) is controversial and not generally accepted. At the moment, there is no cohesive concept of toxin A/B activity to explain all *in vivo* and *in vitro* features.

Both toxin A and toxin B are coexpressed by pathogenic *C. difficile* strains. There are no differences in their intracellular protein targets and only minor differences in enzymic activity. However, the toxins use different cell receptors for cell entry and they show different antigenicity. Thus, both toxins can affect different tissue targets in a sequential way. In addition, the toxins can affect a broad spectrum of hosts from animals to humans by using different cell receptors and by escaping the immunological attack of the host through their diverge antigenicity.

References

1. Wilcox MH. Cleaning up *Clostridium difficile* infection. *Lancet* 1996; 348: 767-8.
2. Kelly CP, Pothoulakis C, LaMont JT. *Clostridium difficile* colitis. *N Engl J Med* 1994; 330 (4): 257-62.
3. Lyerly DM, Krivan HC, Wilkins TD. *Clostridium difficile*: its disease and toxins. *Clin Microbiol Rev* 1988; 1: 1-18.
4. Lyerly DM, Wilkins TD. *Clostridium difficile.* In: Blaser MJ, Smith PD, Ravdin JI, Greenberg HB, Guerrant RL, eds. *Infections of the gastrointestinal tract.* New York: Raven Press, Ltd. 1995: 867-91.
5. Bartlett JG. Management of *Clostridium difficile* infection and other antibiotic-associated diarrhoeas. *Eur J Gastroenterol Hepatol* 1996; 8: 1054-61.
6. Fekety R. Guidelines for the diagnosis and management of *Clostridium difficile*-associated diarrhea and colitis. *Am J Gastroenterol* 1997; 92: 739-50.
7. Borriello SP, Davies HA, Kamiya S, Reed PJ. Virulence factors of *Clostridium difficile. Rev Infect Dis* 1990; 12 (Suppl. 2): 185-91.
8. Sears CL, Kaper JB. Enteric bacterial toxins: Mechanisms of action and linkage to intestinal secretion. *Microbiol Rev* 1996; 60: 167-215.
9. Fiorentini C, Thelestam M. *Clostridium difficile* toxin A and its effects on cells. *Toxicon* 1991; 29: 543-67.
10. Just I, Selzer J, Wilm M, Von Eichel-Streiber C, Mann M, Aktories K. Glucosylation of Rho proteins by *Clostridium difficile* toxin B. *Nature* 1995; 375: 500-3.
11. Just I, Wilm M, Selzer J, *et al.* The enterotoxin from *Clostridium difficile* (ToxA) monoglucosylates the Rho proteins. *J Biol Chem* 1995; 270: 13932-6.
12. Machesky LM, Hall A. Rho: a connection between membrane receptor signalling and the cytoskeleton. *Trends Cell Biol* 1996; 6: 304-10.
13. Narumiya S. The small GTPase Rho: Cellular functions and signal transduction. *J Biochem (Tokyo)* 1996; 120: 215-28.
14. Ridley AJ. Rho: theme and variations. *Curr Biol* 1996; 6: 1256-64.
15. Tapon N, Hall A. Rho, Rac and CDC42 GTPases regulate the organization of the actin cytoskeleton. *Curr Opin Cell Biol* 1997; 9: 86-92.
16. Van Aelst L, D'Souza-Schorey C. Rho GTPases and signaling networks. *Genes Dev* 1997; 11: 2295-322.
17. Hall A. Rho GTPases and the actin cytoskeleton. *Science* 1998; 279: 509-14.
18. Herrmann C, Ahmadian MR, Hofmann F, Just I. Functional consequences of monoglucosylation of H-Ras at effector domain amino acid threonine-35. *J Biol Chem* 1998; in press.
19. Sehr P, Joseph G, Genth H, Just I, Pick E, Aktories K. Glucosylation and ADP-ribosylation of Rho proteins – effects on nucleotide binding, GTPase activity, and effector-coupling. *Biochemistry* 1998; in press.
20. Eichel-Streiber C, Laufenberg-Feldmann R, Sartingen S, Schulze J, Sauerborn M. Comparative sequence analysis of the *Clostridium difficile* toxins A and B. *Mol Gen Genet* 1992; 233: 260-8.

21. Pradel E, Parker CT, Schnaitman CA. Structures of the *rfaB*, *rfaI*, *rfaJ*, and *rfaS* genes of *Escherichia coli* K-12 and their roles in assembly of the lipopolysaccharide core. *J Bacteriol* 1992; 174: 4736-45.
22. Von Eichel-Streiber C, Boquet P, Sauerborn M, Thelestam M. Large clostridial cytotoxins – a family of glycosyltransferases modifying small GTP-binding proteins. *Trends Microbiol* 1996; 375-82.
23. Moncrief JS, Lyerly DM, Wilkins TD. Molecular biology of the *Clostridium difficile* toxins. In: Rood JI, McClane BA, Songer JG, Titball RW, eds. *The clostridia: molecular biology and pathogenesis*. San Diego: Academic Press, 1997: 369-92.
24. Hofmann F, Busch C, Prepens U, Just I, Aktories K. Localization of the glucosyltransferase activity of *Clostridium difficile* toxin B to the N-terminal part of the holotoxin. *J Biol Chem* 1997; 272: 11074-8.
25. Eichel-Streiber C, Sauerborn M. *Clostridium difficile* toxin A carries a C-terminal structure homologous to the carbohydrate binding region of streptococcal glycosyltransferase. *Gene* 1990; 96: 107-13.
26. Pothoulakis C, Gilbert RJ, Cladaras C, *et al.* Rabbit sucrase-isomaltase contains a functional intestinal receptor for *Clostridium difficile* toxin A. *J Clin Invest* 1996; 98: 641-9.
27. Aktories K, Just I. Monoglucosylation of low-molecular-mass GTP-binding Rho proteins by clostridial cytotoxins. *Trends Cell Biol* 1995; 5: 441-3.
28. Aktories K. Rho proteins: targets for bacterial toxins. *Trends Microbiol* 1997; 5: 282-8.
29. Boquet P, Munro P, Fiorentini C, Just I. Toxins from anaerobic bacteria: specificity and molecular mechanisms of action. *Curr Opin Microbiol* 1998; 1: 66-74.
30. Pothoulakis C, LaMont JT, Eglow R, *et al.* Charaterizing of rabbit ileal receptors for *Clostridium difficile* toxin A. *J Clin Invest* 1991; 88: 119-25.
31. Pothoulakis C, Galili U, Castagliuolo I, *et al.* A human antibody binds to a-galactose receptors and mimics the effects of *Clostridium difficile* toxin A in rat colon. *Gastroenterology* 1996; 110: 1704-12.

Recent advances in the pathogenesis of gastrointestinal bacterial infections.
P. Rampal, P. Boquet, eds. John Libbey Eurotext, Paris © 1998, pp. 143-153.

Shiga and Shiga-like toxins

Sjur Olsnes

Institute for Cancer Research, The Norwegian Radium Hospital, Montebello, 031 Oslo, Norway

Shiga toxin was first identified as a toxic protein produced by the most virulent *Shigella* species, *Shigella dysenteriae* type 1. The toxin is not produced by other pathogenic *Shigella* strains and it is believed to be the cause for the much higher lethality of infections with *S. dysenteriae* than with other *Shigella* strains (for review [1]).

The first evidence that *S. dysenteriae* produces a toxin was obtained by Conradi [2] who discovered that small amounts of sterile filtrates of *S. dysenteriae* cause paralysis, diarrhoea and death when injected intravenously into rabbits. With improving purification techniques increasing specific activity of the preparations were obtained. van Heyningen and Gladstone [3] obtained a highly purified preparation that led them to conclude that Shiga toxin is one of the most active toxins known. They found that the toxin was toxic to tissue cultures as well as to whole animals. Due to the different symptoms observed in intoxicated animals, it was for a long time discussed whether there exists one or three different toxins, an enterotoxic, a cytotoxic and a neurotoxic component. With pure toxin it could finally be demonstrated that the different activities are due to one toxin [4] and that its primary target is the endothelium [1].

As soon as the Shiga toxin had been identified and characterized [5], search for related toxins in other bacterial species was initiated [1]. Certain strains of enteropathogenic *Escherichia coli*, particularly those belonging to serotype O157:H7, proved to express identical or similar toxins (Shiga-like toxins, SLT-I and SLT-II, also called Verotoxins, because they were first found to be toxic to Vero cells). These strains were found to be associated with haemolytic uraemic syndrome (HUS) [6]. This disease is characterized by a prodroma of non-febrile gastroenteritis, often with bloody stools, which is followed by microangiopathic hemolytic anaemia, thrombocytopenia and uraemia [7] is an increasingly common reason for renal failure requiring renal transplantation [8]. The syndrome is characterized by lack of fever and with wide-spread sterile lesions characterized by microangiopathic lesions in

kidney and other organs. The disease is also observed after infections with *S. dysenteriae* type 1. *E. coli* serotype O157:H7 is found with increasing frequency in the bovine intestine and it often contaminates beef due to improper handling in the slaughterhouse. Infection of humans from insufficiently heated beef is therefore an increasing problem. The disease occurs preferentially in children and in elderly people. Thrombotic thrombocytopenic purpura is another syndrome associated with *E. coli* serotype 0157:H7 and is probably due to the same toxin [9].
The edema disease of piglet, which is characterized by edema, perivascular hemorhage and necrosis of small blood vessels is due to a related toxin (SLT-IIe). In this disease the lesions are primarily in the submucosa of the stomach and colon, in the colonic mesentery, the eyelids and the cerebellum [10].

Characterization of Shiga and SLT toxins and their relation to plant toxins

Shiga toxin and SLT-1 and SLT-2 consist of two functionally different subunits, termed A and B *(figure 1)* [11]. The A-subunit consists of a single polypeptide chain (32 kD) which contains a protease-sensitive, disulfide-bridged loop in its C-terminal end *(figure 2)*. The loop contains a site sensitive for the trans-Golgi protease furin [12], and it can also be cleaved by trypsin [11]. The A-chain contains enzymatic activity that is activated upon cleavage of the loop and reduction of the disulfide to liberate the larger A_1-fragment [11, 13, 14]. The A_2-fragment is bound non-covalently to the B-subunit. The B-subunit consists of a pentamer of 7.7-kD proteins that are formed like a ring [15, 16]. The function of the B-subunit is to bind the toxin to receptors at the cell surface and guide the toxin to the location in the cell where the enzymatically active A_1-fragment can cross the membrane and enter the cytosol.

Shiga toxin was cloned simultaneously in two laboratories [17, 18]. As soon as the sequence became available, it appeared that the A-subunit showed strong homology to a plant toxin, ricin [17-19]. There was no homology between the B-subunits of the two toxins. As will be discussed below, the A-subunits of ricin and Shiga toxin have the same intracellular target.

Analysis of the crystal structure of Shiga toxin demonstrated that the five B-subunits are organised as a ring encircling a helix at the carboxyterminus of the A_2 fragment [16]. Each B-chain is folded into one α-helix and six β-strands. The α-helix is located inside the peptameric ring and the β-strands form antiparallel β-sheets on the outside of the pentameric ring. The C-terminal helix of the A-subunit is oriented antiparallel to the 5 α-helices of the B-chain. The A_1-fragment is located on top of the pentameric ring. The fold of the A subunit is similar to that of ricin A-chain [16]. Part of the A_2-fragment is located in the active site of the A_1-fragment and may deny access of the substrate. The structure of Shiga toxin B subunit resembles that of cholera toxin, but the A subunits are different. The disulfide bond between the A_1- and A_2-fragments is required to keep the nicked toxin together. Thus, when Cys242 was mutated to Ser, such that a disulfide bond could not be formed, the A_1-fragment was released from the toxin as soon as the A-subunit was cleaved [20].

The SLT of enteropathogenic *E. coli* of subtype O157:H2 and others closely resemble Shiga toxin. Whereas the Shiga toxin gene appears to be at the chromosome, the SLT toxins are encoded by lysogenic phages [21]. SLT-1 is identical with Shiga toxin at the amino acid level except for one amino acid, whereas SLT-2 is more different [22].

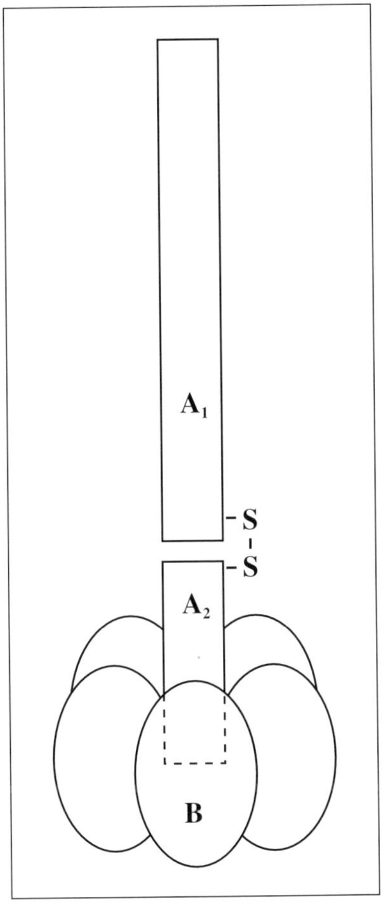

Figure 1. Schematic structure of cleaved Shiga toxin. The toxin consists of an A-subunit which is cleaved into the A_1 and A_2 fragments that are linked by a disulfide bridge. The A_2-fragment is associated with the b-subunit, which is a pentameric ring of identical B-chains.

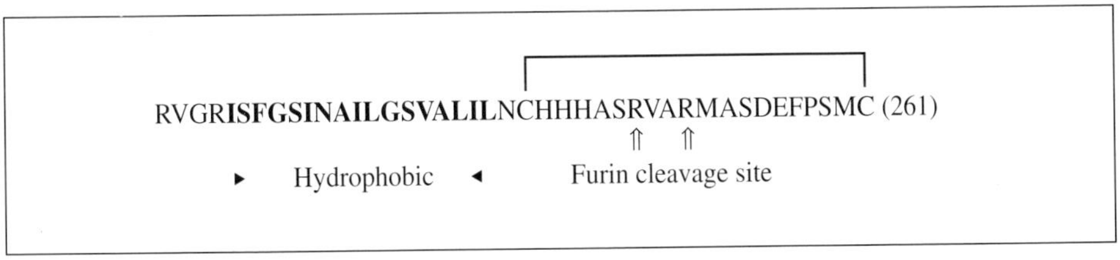

Figure 2. Amino acid sequence of the hydrophobic region of the A-chain and the disulfide-bridged loop with the furin cleavage site. When the A-chain is cleaved by furin or trypsin, the appearing A_1-fragment has a C-terminal hydrophobic sequence indicated here with bold face. The disulfide keeps the cleaved A-chain together, but upon reduction, the A_1-fragment is released.

Interaction with cells

Shiga toxin and SLT toxins have a strong preference for endothelial cells. Soon after their isolation, search was therefore carried out for the cellular receptor for the toxins. The first studies demonstrated that some cells are binding large amounts of the toxins whereas others are not binding measurable amounts [23]. Furthermore, many cells that bound much toxin were found to be resistant to the toxic effect.

Further search for the receptor demonstrated that the glycolipid fraction was most efficient in toxin binding and it eventually was found that CD77 [24-26], the glycolipid globotriaosyl ceramide (Gb_3), is the functional receptor for Shiga toxin, SLT-I and SLT-II. Incorporation of Gb_3 into Daudi cells that lack receptors resulted in sensitization of the cells to the toxin [27]. Human umbilical vein endothelial cells have normally low levels of Gb_3, but upon treatment with tumor necrosis factor-α or bacterial lipopolysaccharides they increased the expression of Gb_3 4-6 fold and became toxin sensitive [28].

Gb_3 is a large fraction of human renal glycolipids [29]. Gb_3 is the P^k antigen of the P blood group and identical to CD77 [24], but the toxins do not bind to erythrocytes [30]. Digalactosyl-diglyceride has the same carbohydrate group as Gb_3, but it lacks the ceramide part and showed no ability to bind Shiga toxin [31]. Two cell surface proteins, CD19 and interferon-γ receptor have considerable sequence homology with Shiga toxin B-subunit [24].

SLT-IIe which induces the edema disease in piglets is closely related to SLT-II in structure, but it binds to a separate glycolipid, Gb_4 that is not recognized by the other toxins here described [10]. Cells lacking Gb_4 are resistant to SLT-IIe. Targeted mutagenesis of defined amino acids in the toxin B-subunit was able to convert the specificity of SLT-IIe to that of SLT-II, *i.e.* the toxin lost affinity for Gb_4 and gained affinity for Gb_3 [32].

Endocytosis and vesicular transport

Electron microscopic studies demonstrated that Shiga toxin binds to the entire cell surface membrane, but upon incubation at 37° C it was rapidly transported to coated pits and endocytosed [33]. A considerable amount of the endocytosed toxin was later found in the *trans*-Golgi network *(figure 3)*.

It had been observed that when A431 cells that are resistant to Shiga toxin were treated with butyric acid, they became sensitive to the toxin [34]. Interestingly, in polarized MDCK cells funtional receptors were induced both on the basolateral and apical side. Ultrastructural analysis of such cells treated with a conjugate of Shiga toxin and horse radish peroxidase showed that in the butyrate-treated cells a considerable amount of the conjugate was transported retrograde to the endoplasmic reticulum (ER) including the perinuclear space [35]. This was the first observation of an extracellularly added protein that is transported retrograde through the Golgi apparatus to the ER. Treatments that increased the level of intracellular cAMP had an effect similar to that of butyric acid [36].

The isolated B-subunit of Shiga toxin was also transported retrograde to the ER in butytic acid treated A431 cells [36]. The ceramide moiety of the Gb_3 in the butyric acid treated cells had longer fatty acids that in the untreated cells, indicating that te fatty acid composition is important for retrograde transport [36].

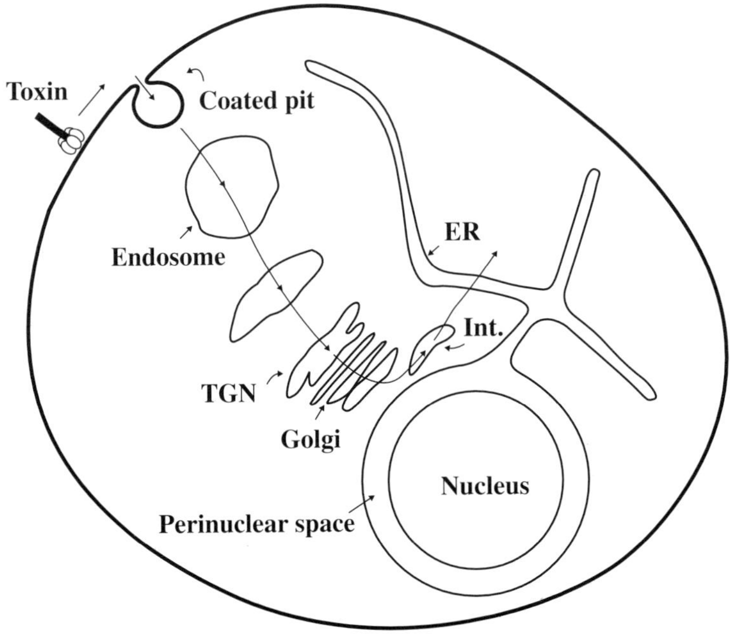

Figure 3. Schematic indication of the intracellular routing of Shiga toxin. The toxin binds to Gb_3 at the cell sulface and is then rapidly transported to coated pits. The coated pits pinch off, loose their clathrin coat and fuse with endosomes. The toxin is then transported retrograde to the *trans*-Golgi network (TGN), through the Golgi stacks, to the intermediary compartment (Int.) and finally to the endoplasmic reticulum (ER). The toxin A_1-fragment appears to be translocated across the membrane of the ER to reach its target, the ribosomal 28S RNA.

That retrograde transport of a toxin to the ER may be necessary for penetration to the cytosol was first proposed by Chaudhary *et al.* [37]. They noted that two toxins that act in the cytosol, cholera toxin and *E. coli* heat-labile toxin contain in the C-terminal end of their A-subunits a KDEL and RDEL sequence, respectively. These sequences are present on resident ER lumen proteins and they are required for retrieval of luminal ER proteins in the intermediary compartment and in the Golgi apparatus due to binding to the KDEL-receptor located here. Thus they ensure that the proteins are not exported out of the cells. The finding of KDEL and RDEL sequences in two bacterial toxins (bacteria do not have proteins that bind the sequence) strongly suggested that the toxins are guided to the ER. Chaudhary *et al.* [37] found that exotoxin A from *Pseudomonas aeruginosa* contains a similar sequence in its C-terminus, RDELK. The terminal lysine residue has later been found to be easily removed by cellular exopeptidases, leaving the RDEL sequence that is able to bind to the KDEL receptor. They found that when they removed or mutated the sequence, the toxin lost activity and that the activity was restored when they added a KDEL sequence instead.

It should be noted that Shiga and SLT do not contain a KDEL or a related sequence. Their retrograde transport must therefore rely on binding to other molecules that guide them to the ER. Addition of a KDEL sequence to Shiga toxin B-subunit increased the amount of B-subunit in the ER, whereas addition of the non-functional KDELGL sequence resulted in more of the B-subunit being transported back to the Golgi region [38]. Glycosylation of a N-glycosylation site engineered into the B-subunit occurred at the same rate in both cases, indicating that the rate of transport from the cell surface to the ER was not influenced by the presence of the KDEL sequence [38].

Also ricin does not contain a KDEL-like sequence. Since it has an enzymatically active A-chain that resembles that of Shiga toxin, it was interesting to study if also this toxin is transported retrograde to the ER. It had been known for some time that ricin is transported to the *trans*-Golgi network [39], but ultrastructural analysis could not reveal transport to the ER. Therefore the toxin was modified to contain a tyrosine sulfation signal that allows it to be labelled with radioactive sulfate when it is transported from the exterior to the Golgi apparatus [40]. The toxin A-chain was also modified to contain glysosylation sites to allow detection of molecules that had reached the ER. It was found that the major part of the toxin that had reached the Golgi apparatus and become labelled with sulfate was also transported to the ER where it became glycosylated. Addition of a KDEL sequence to the C-terminal end of ricin A-chain increased the rate of transport from the Golgi apparatus to the ER.

Penetration to the cytosol

It is not known how Shiga toxin or SLT penetrate the membrane, but the translocation is believed to take place in the ER. Experiments with ricin support this hypothesis. Ricin modified as discussed above was found to be translocated to the cytosol in the glycosylated form [40]. This indicates that only molecules that had reached the ER are translocated. So far the translocation mechanism as such is not known, but a tempting hypothesis is that the protein is translocated by the Sec61p system, *i.e.* by reversal or the transport of export proteins from the cytosol to the ER. The translocation could be guided by a hydrophobic amino acid stretch that is located close to the C-terminus of the A-chains of abrin and ricin, and close to the C-terminus of the A_1 fragments of Shiga *(figure 2)* and SLT toxins [41]. In the case of ricin, this sequence, when fused to the N-terminal end of dihydrofolate reductase, was able to target this normally cytosolic enzyme into microsomes [42]. Furthermore, a mutation in this region reduced the toxicity of ricin [43].

There is an increasing amount of information that such retrograde translocation can occur. Thus it has recently been observed that the extensive degradation of misfolded proteins earlier believed to take place in the ER does not occur within the lumen. Rather, the proteins are translocated back into the cytosol where they are degraded by a process involving proteasomes [44-47]. The degradation can be inhibited with proteasome inhibitors. Possibly, the toxins are recognized as misfolded proteins in the ER and then translocated to the cytosol.

If this is so, the toxins must somehow avoid the proteasomes. In the case of ricin the ability to escape degradation by proteasomes is only partial, and the toxin is more active and survives longer in the cytosol when the cells are incubated in the presence of inhibitors of proteasomes (unpublished data).

It is not clear if the A-chain of Shiga and SLT toxins must be cleaved to yield A_1 and A_2 fragments before translocation can occur. Thus, three groups have presented evidence that mutated toxin that cannot be cleaved by furin or trypsin is highly toxic [12, 48, 49].

Molecular mode of action

Once inside the cells the toxins inactivate the ribosomes and thereby block protein synthesis [13]. The enzymatic activity is contained in the A_1-fragment of Shiga and SLT toxins [14] which are N-glycosidases that recognise a single adenosine residue that is located close to the 3' end of the 28 S ribosomal RNA [50]. The toxin removes the adenine at this position without breaking the phosphosugar backbone of the RNA. This adenine residue is involved in the binding of elongation factors to the ribosomes and the toxin-treated ribosomes are therefore unable to continue protein synthesis. A large number of plant proteins, including the toxins abrin and ricin, have the same enzymatic activity as Shiga and SLT toxins [51, 52].

Applications

Since Shiga and Shiga-like toxins are of widespread concern as etiology for serious diseases both in developing ad industrialized countries, considerable effort is being made to develop vaccines against the toxigenic bacteria and against the toxins as such [53]. The edema disease in piglets has been extensively used in such studies, both because prevention of the disease is of economic importance and because it can be used as an animal model system to study prevention of the human diseases. Both vaccines based on a toxoid [54] and on a toxin molecule mutated at a critical site in the enzymatically active site in the A-subunit [55] have given promising results.

A possible use of the active toxin in cancer therapy has been considered. SLT-1 appears to be the active compound in a bacteriocin preparation from *E. coli* that has been demonstrated to be active against human ovarian cancer cells in culture and when the cells were grown as tumors in mice. The ovarian tumors and metastases were found to contain high levels of Gb_3 [56].

The B-subunit of Shiga and SLT toxins can be used to target molecules to the Golgi apparatus and even to the ER. B-subunit of SLT-1 labelled with fluorescein, which emits light in a pH-dependent way, was used to probe the pH of the Golgi apparatus [57]. It was found that the pH inside the Golgi apparatus was 6.45 ± 0.03. The pH increased rapidly upon treatment with bafilomycin A_1, an inhibitor of the vascular type proton pump. The possibility of using the B-subunit to target drugs and proteins to the Golgi apparatus and to the ER is being considered.

References

1. O'Brien AD, Holmes RK. Shiga and Shiga-like toxins. *Microbiol Rev* 1987; 51: 206-20.
2. Conradi H. Ueber lösliche, durch aseptische Autolyse erhaltene Giftstoffe von Ruhr- und Typhusbacillen. *Dtsch Med Wochenschr* 1903; 20: 26-8.
3. Van Heyningen WE, Gladstone GP. The neurotoxin of *Shigella Shigae*. 1. Production, purification and properties of the toxin. *Br J Exp Pathol* 1953; 34: 202-16.
4. Eiklid K, Olsnes S. Animal toxicity of *Shigella dysenteriae* cytotoxin: evidence that the neurotoxic, enterotoxic, and cytotoxic activities are due to one toxin. *J Immunol* 1983; 130: 380-4.
5. Olsnes S, Eiklid K. Isolation and characterization of *Shigella shigae* cytotoxin. *J Biol Chem* 1980; 255: 284-9.
6. Karmali MA, Steele BT, Petric M, Lim C. Sporadic cases of haemolytic-uraemic syndrome associated with faecal cytotoxin and cytotoxin-producing *Escherichia coli* in stools. *Lancet* 1983; 1: 619-20.
7. Gasser C, Gautier E, Steck A, Siebenmann RE, Oeschlin R. Hämolytisch-urämische Syndrome: Bilaterale Nierenrindennekrosen bei akuten erworbenen Anämien. *Schweiz Med Wochenschr* 1955; 85: 905-9.
8. Kavi J, Wise R. Causes of the haemolytic uraemic syndrome. *Br Med J* 1989; 298: 65-6.
9. Ashkenazi S. Role of bacterial cytotoxins in hemolytic uremic syndrome and thrombotic thrombocytopenic purpura. *Annu Rev Med* 1993; 44: 11-8.
10. DeGrandis S, Law H, Brunton J, Gyles C, Lingwood CA. Globotetraosylceramide is recognized by the pig edema disease toxin. *J Biol Chem* 1989; 264: 12520-5.
11. Olsnes S, Reisbig R, Eiklid K. Subunit structure of *Shigella* cytotoxin. *J Biol Chem* 1981; 256: 8732-8.
12. Garred O, Dubinina E, Holm PK, Olsnes S, van Deurs B, Kozlov JV, Sandvig K. Role of processing and intracellular transport for optimal toxicity of Shiga toxin and toxin mutants. *Exp Cell Res* 1995; 218: 39-49.
13. Brown JE, Ussery MA, Leppla SH, Rothman SW. Inhibition of protein synthesis by Shiga toxin: activation of the toxin and inhibition of peptide elongation. *FEBS Lett* 1980; 117: 84-8.
14. Reisbig R, Olsnes S, Eiklid K. The cytotoxic activity of *Shigella* toxin. Evidence for catalytic inactivation of the 60 S ribosomal subunit. *J Biol Chem* 1981; 256: 8739-44.
15. Stein PE, Boodhoo A, Tyrrell GJ, Brunton JL, Read RJ. Crystal structure of the cell-binding B oligomer of verotoxin-1 from *E. coli*. *Nature* 1992; 355: 748-50.
16. Fraser ME, Chernaia MM, Kozlov YV, James MN. Crystal structure of the holotoxin from *Shigella dysenteriae* at 2.5 A resolution. *Nat Struct Biol* 1994; 1: 59-64.

17. Kozlov YuV, Kabishev AA, Lukyanov EV, Bayev AA. The primary structure of the operons coding for *Shigella dysenteriae* toxin and temperature phage H30 shiga-like toxin. *Gene* 1998; 67: 213-21.
18. Calderwood SB, Auclair F, Donohue-Rolfe A, Keusch GT, Mekalanos JJ. Nucleotide sequence of the Shiga-like toxin genes of *Escherichia coli. Proc Natl Acad Sci USA* 1987; 84: 4364-8.
19. Olsnes S. Closing in on ricin action. *Nature* 1987; 328: 474-5.
20. Garred O, Dubinina E, Polesskaya A, Olsnes S, Kozlov J, Sandvig K. Role of the disulfide bond in Shiga toxin A-chain for toxin entry into cells. *J Biol Chem* 1998; 272: 11414-9.
21. Strockbine NA, Marques LR, Newland JW, Smith HW, Holmes RK, O'Brien AD. Two toxin-converting phages from *Escherichia coli* O157:H7 strain 933 encode antigenically distinct toxins with similar biologic activities. *Infect Immun* 1998; 53: 135-40.
22. Ito H, Terai A, Kurazono H, Takeda Y, Nishibuchi M. Cloning and nucleotide sequencing of Vero toxin 2 variant genes from *Escherichia coli* O91:H21 isolated from a patient with the hemolytic uremic syndrome [published erratum appears in *Microb Pathog* 8: 449]. *Microb Pathog* 1990; 8: 47-60.
23. Eiklid K, Olsnes S. Interaction of *Shigella shigae* cytotoxin with receptors on sensitive and insensitive cells. *J Recept Res* 1980; 1: 199-213.
24. Maloney MD, Lingwood CA. CD19 has a potential CD77 (globotriaosyl ceramide)-binding site with sequence similarity to verotoxin B-subunits: implications of molecular mimicry for B cell adhesion and enterohemorrhagic *Escherichia coli* pathogenesis. *J Exp Med* 1994; 180: 191-201.
25. Lindberg AA, Brown JE, Strømberg N, Wesling-Ryd M, Schultz JE, Karlsson KA, Stromberg N, Westling-Ryd M. Identification of the carbohydrate receptor for Shiga toxin produced by *Shigella dysenteriae* Type 1. *J Biol Chem* 1987; 262: 1779-85.
26. Jacewicz M, Clausen H, Nudelman E, Donohue-Rolfe A, Keusch GT. Pathogenesis of *Shigella diarrhea*. XI. Isolation of a *Shigella* toxin-binding glycolipid from rabbit jejunum and HeLa cells and its identification as globotriasylceramide. *J Exp Med* 1986; 163: 1391-404.
27. Waddell T, Cohen A, Lingwood CA. Induction of verotoxin sensitivity in receptor-deficient cell lines using the receptor glycolipid globotriosylceramide. *Proc Natl Acad Sci USA* 1990; 87: 7898-901.
28. Obrig TG, Louise CB, Lingwood CA, Boyd B, Barley-Maloney L, Daniel TO. Endothelial heterogeneity in Shiga toxin receptors and responses. *J Biol Chem* 1993; 268: 15484-8.
29. Lingwood CA. Verotoxin-binding in human renal sections. *Nephron* 1994; 66: 21-8.
30. Calvete JA, Newell DR, Wright AF, Rose MS. *In vitro* and *in vivo* antitumor activity of ZENECA ZD0490, a recombinant ricin A-chain immunotoxin for the treatment of colorectal cancer. *Cancer Res* 1994; 54: 4684-90.
31. Lingwood CA, Law H, Richardson S, Petric M, Brunton JL, De Grandis S, Karmali M. Glycolipid binding of purified and recombinant *Escherichia coli* produced verotoxin *in vitro*. *J Biol Chem* 1987; 262: 8834-9.
32. Tyrrell GJ, Ramotar K, Toye B, Boyd B, Lingwood CA, Brunton JL. Alteration of the carbohydrate binding specificity of verotoxins from Galα1-4Gal to GalNAcβ1-3Galα1-4Gal and vice versa by site-directed mutagenesis of the binding subunit. *Proc Natl Acad Sci USA* 1992; 89: 524-8.
33. Sandvig K, Olsnes S, Brown JE, Petersen OW, van Deurs B. Endocytosis from coated pits of Shiga toxin: a glycolipid-binding protein from *Shigella dysenteriae 1. J Cell Biol* 1989; 108: 1331-43.
34. Sandvig K, Prydz K, Ryd M, van Deurs B. Endocytosis and intracellular transport of the glycolipid-binding ligand Shiga toxin in polarized MDCK cells. *J Cell Biol* 1991; 113: 553-62.

35. Sandvig K, Garred O, Prydz K, Kozlov JV, Hansen SH, van Deurs B. Retrograde transport of endocytosed Shiga toxin to the endoplasmic reticulum. *Nature* 1992; 358: 510-2.
36. Sandvig K, Ryd M, Garred O, Schweda E, Holm PK, van Deurs B. Retrograde transport from the Golgi complex to the ER of both Shiga toxin and the nontoxic Shiga B-fragment is regulated by butyric acid and cAMP. *J Cell Biol* 1998; 126: 53-64.
37. Chaudhary VK, Jinno Y, FitzGerald D, Pastan I. Pseudomonas exotoxin contains a specific sequence at the carboxyl terminus that is required for cytotoxicity. *Proc Natl Acad Sci USA* 1990; 87: 308-12.
38. Johannes L, Tenza D, Antony C, Goud B. Retrograde transport of KDEL-bearing B-fragment of Shiga toxin. *J Biol Chem* 1998; 272: 19554-61.
39. Van Deurs B, T:nnessen TI, Petersen OW, Sandvig K, Olsnes S. Routing of internalized ricin and ricin conjugates to the Golgi complex. *J Cell Biol* 1986; 102: 37-47.
40. Rapak A, Falnes PO, Olsnes S. Retrograde transport of mutant ricin to the endoplasmic reticulum with subsequent translocation to cytosol. *Proc Natl Acad Sci USA* 1998; 94: 3783-8.
41. Saleh MT, Ferguson J, Boggs JM, Gariepy J. Insertion and orientation of a synthetic peptide representing the C-terminus of the A_1 domain of Shiga toxin into phospholipid membranes. *Biochemistry* 1998; 35: 9325-34.
42. Chaddock JA, Roberts LM, Jungnickel B, Lord JM. A hydrophobic region of ricin A chain which may have a role in membrane translocation can function as an efficient noncleaved signal peptide. *Biochem Biophys Res Commun* 1998; 217: 68-73.
43. Simpson JC, Lord JM, Roberts LM. Point mutations in the hydrophobic C-terminal region of ricin A chain indicate that Pro250 plays a key role in membrane translocation. *Eur J Biochem* 1998; 232: 458-63.
44. Knop M, Finger A, Braun T, Hellmuth K, Wolf DH. Der1, a novel protein specifically required for endoplasmic reticulum degradation in yeast. *EMBO J* 1996; 15: 753-63.
45. Hiller M, Finger A, Schweiger M, Wolf D. ER degradation of a misfolded luminal protein by the cytosolic ubiquitin-proteasome pathway. *Science* 1996; 273: 1725-8.
46. Werner ED, Brodsky JL, McCracken AA. Proteasome-dependent endoplasmic reticulum-associated protein degradation: an unconventional route to a familiar fate. *Proc Natl Acad Sci USA* 1996; 93: 13797-801.
47. Wiertz EJ, Jones TR, Sun L, Bogyo M, Geuze HJ, Ploegh HL. The human cytomegalovirus US11 gene product dislocates MHC class I heavy chains from the endoplasmic reticulum to the cytosol. *Cell* 1996; 84: 769-79.
48. Burgess BJ, Roberts LM. Proteolytic cleavage at arginine residues within the hydrophilic disulphide loop of the *Escherichia coli* Shiga-like toxin I A subunit is not essential for cytotoxicity. *Mol Microbiol* 1993; 10: 171-9.
49. Samuel JE, Gordon VM. Evidence that proteolytic separation of Shiga-like toxin type IIv A subunit into A_1 and A_2 subunits is not required for toxin activity. *J Biol Chem* 1994; 269: 4853-9.
50. Endo Y, Tsurugi K, Yutsudo T, Takeda Y, Ogasawara T, Igarashi K. Site of action of a Vero toxin (VT2) from *Escherichia coli* O157:H7 and of Shiga toxin on eukaryotic ribosomes. RNA N-glycosidase activity of the toxins. *Eur J Biochem* 1988; 171: 45-50.
51. Endo Y, Mitsui K, Motizuki M, Tsurugi K. The mechanism of action of ricin and related toxic lectins on eukaryotic ribosomes. The site and the characteristics of the modification in 28 S ribosomal RNA caused by the toxins. *J Biol Chem* 1987; 262: 5908-12.
52. Endo Y, Tsurugi K. RNA N-glycosidase activity of ricin A-chain. Mechanism of action of the toxic lectin ricin on eukaryotic ribosomes. *J Biol Chem* 1987; 262: 8128-30.
53. Arnon R. Synthetic vaccines based on peptides, oligonucleotides and conjugate antigens. *Behring Inst Mitt* 1998; 184-90.

54. Johansen M, Andresen LO, Jorsal SE, Thomsen LK, Waddell TE, Gyles CL. Prevention of edema disease in pigs by vaccination with verotoxin 2e toxoid. *Can J Vet Res* 1998; 61: 280-5.
55. Gordon VM, Whipp SC, Moon HW, O'Brien AD, Samuel JE. An enzymatic mutant of Shiga-like toxin II variant is a vaccine candidate for edema disease of swine. *Infect Immun* 1998; 60: 485-90.
56. Farkas-Himsley H, Hill R, Rosen B, Arab S, Lingwood CA. The bacterial colicin active against tumor cells *in vitro* and *in vivo* is verotoxin 1. *Proc Natl Acad Sci USA* 1995; 92: 6996-7000.
57. Kim JH, Lingwood CA, Williams DB, Furuya W, Manolson MF, Grinstein S. Dynamic measurement of the pH of the golgi complex in living cells using retrograde transport of the verotoxin receptor. *J Cell Biol* 1996; 134: 1387-99.

Recent advances in the pathogenesis of gastrointestinal bacterial infections.
P. Rampal, P. Boquet, eds. John Libbey Eurotext, Paris © 1998, pp. 155-164.

Cholera toxin B subunit as transmucosal carrier-delivery and immunomodulating system for induction of anti-infectious and anti-pathological immunity

Cecil Czerkinsky

INSERM Unité 64, Nice, France, and Department of Medical Microbiology and Immunology, Göteborg University, Sweden

Mucosal surfaces represent the largest organ system in vertebrates. Being the most frequent portals of entry of common microbes and environmental antigens, these surfaces provide a critical barrier against entry of exogenous matters. Endowed with powerful mechanical and physicochemical cleansing mechanisms, these surfaces are further protected by a specialized immune system that guards them against potential insults from the environment.

The gut-associated lymphoid tissue (GALT), the largest mammalian lymphoid organ system, represents a well known example of compartmentalized immunological system as evidenced by (i) the existence of defined lymphoid microcompartments within the gut, (ii) phenotypically and functionally distinct B-cell, T-cell, and accessory cell subpopulations, and (iii) restrictions imposed upon lymphoid cell recirculation potential to (and from) the gut or even within various regions of the intestine [1]. Through the compartmentalization of its afferent and efferent limbs, the GALT functions essentially independently from the systemic immune apparatus, at least as regard induction of humoral immune responses. This notion explains why systemic injection of immunogens is relatively ineffective at inducing an antibody response in the intestinal mucosa.

The GALT has three main functions: to protect against colonization and invasion by the large number of potentially dangerous microbes, to prevent uptake of undegraded antigens including foreign proteins derived from ingested food and commensal microorganisms, and to prevent the development of potentially harmful immune responses to these antigens. At variance with the systemic immune apparatus, which is a sterile compartment and can respond vigourously to most invaders, the GALT guards tissues that are replete with foreign matters including microorganisms and dietary products. It follows that upon encounter with a given antigen, the GALT must select appropriate effector mechanisms and regulate the intensity of its response so as to avoid by-stander tissue damage and immunological exhaustion.

Mucosal vaccines

Immune responses expressed in mucosal tissues are typified by secretory immunoglobulin A (SIgA), the predominant Ig class in human external secretions (and by far the most abundant class of antibodies in this species), and the best known entity providing specific immune protection for mucosal tissues [1]. SIgA antibodies provide "immune exclusion" of bacterial and viral pathogens, bacterial toxins and other potentially harmful molecules, and have also been reported to neutralize directly a number of viruses, to mediate antibody-dependent cell-mediated cytotoxicity (in cooperation with macrophages, lymphocytes and eosinophils), and to interfere with the utilization of growth factors for bacterial pathogens in the mucosal environment [1]. Interestingly, SIgA not only functions well in external secretions but also can express its antimicrobial properties within the epithelial cell, that is the very same cell that transport newly formed IgA molecules from the subepithelial lymphoid compartment to the external side of a mucosal tissue. Furthermore, being devoid of complement-activating properties and relatively inefficient as opsonin, SIgA represents a unique type of non-inflammatory specific immune effector molecule.

Based on the concept of a common mucosal immune system through which a fraction of IgA-committed B cells recruited in the gut, *e.g.* by ingestion of antigen, can disseminate immunity not only in the intestine but also to other mucosal and glandular tissues, there is currently much interest in the possiblity to develop oral vaccines against, *e.g.* infections in the buccal, occular, respiratory and genital mucosae.

In addition to SIgA antibody formation, cytotoxicity mediated by T lymphocytes (CTL), antibody-dependent cytotoxicity, and natural killer activity can develop in mucosal tissues, especially in the epithelium of the gastrointestinal tract [2-4]. Oral administration of allogeneic cells and viruses has been shown to induce specific CTLs in Peyer's patches and other mucosal tissues [5]. Because CTLs are critical for eliminating virus-infected cells, their presence in the epithelium of mucosal tissues and their potential role as a first line of defense against invasion by viruses should be advantageous to the host, a possibility that deserves being investigated more thoroughly.

It is now almost axiomatic that in order to be efficacious, vaccines against mucosal infections must stimulate the mucosal immune system, and that this goal is usually better achieved by administering immunogens by the oral route rather than parenterally. However, stimulation of mucosal immune responses by *e.g.* the oral consumption, inhalation or topical deposition of most non-viable antigens is often inefficient, requiring multiple administrations of large (milligram to gram) quantities of immunogens and yielding, if any, modest and short-lasting antibody responses. It has thus been widely assumed that only live vaccines would efficiently stimulate a mucosal immune response. The use of live attenuated recombinant bacteria and viruses which can be genetically engineered to express unrelated antigens is being advocated since natural infection with live microorganisms is known to induce persistent and strong immune responses in both mucosal and systemic compartments. However, with most live microbial vectors, a critical balance between attenuation, adequate expression, and immunogenicity is often difficult to achieve, and potential side effects associated with tissue-damaging DTH-like reactions can.

Alternative strategies of antigen delivery include liposomes, biodegradable microspheres such as copolymers of poly DL-lactide-co-glycolide, polyphosphacenes, polyalginates, cellulose starch with incorporated or surface-adsorbed antigens have been utilized but their preparation generally requires relatively large amounts of antigens and/or harsh conditions resulting in potential denaturation of antigens. Mucosal lectin-like molecules endowed with immunostimulatory properties, such as cholera toxin (CT), the most potent mucosal immunogen and adjuvant known so far, and its analog *Escherishia coli* heat-labile enterotoxin (LT), when coadministered with either unconjugated or conjugated antigens have been shown to promote mucosal and systemic antibody responses. This is due to a large extent to the ability of cholera toxin to bind avidly to GM1 ganglioside on cell surfaces including epithelial M cells, a property ascribed to its B subunit, and to another extent to the adjuvant properties of the toxin which appear to require the ADP-ribosylating action of the enterotoxic A subunit [6].

Oral tolerance

Mucosal uptake of Ag has far more ensuing consequences than systemic intake of Ag on the development of immune responsiveness. Not only can it induce secretory IgA antibody responses in various mucosal tissues but also, and often, systemic tolerance, or even both. Induction of either or both types of responses could be advantageous to protect the host from colonization by mucosal pathogens and from pathogenic systemic responses that may develop against absorbed Ag produced by these pathogens.

Mucosal administration of antigens is in fact a long-recognized method of inducing peripheral tolerance [7]. The phenomenon, often referred to as "oral tolerance" (because initially documented by the effect of oral administration of Ag), is characterized by the fact that animals fed or having inhaled an antigen become refractory or have diminished capability to develop an immune response when re-exposed to that very same Ag introduced by the systemic route, *e.g.* by injection. This phenomenon is an important natural physiological mechanism whereby we avoid to develop DTH reactions to many ingested food proteins and other antigens [8]. Depending upon the dose of antigen administered, anergy of antigen-specific T cells, clonal deletion of proinflammatory T cells, and/or expansion of cells producing immunosuppressive cytokines (IL-4, IL-10 and TGF-β) may result in decreased T cell immune responsiveness [9]. It is interesting to note that the latter scenario involves cytokines that are also known to up-regulate IgA production [1, 10] and is thus compatible with the observation that secretory humoral immune responses and systemic T cell tolerance may develop concommittantly [11]. Because tolerance can be transferred by both serum and cells from tolerized animals, it is possible that humoral antibodies (IgA?), circulating undegraded antigens or tolerogenic fragments and cytokines may act synergistically to confer T cell unresponsiveness. Since mucosally-induced immunological tolerance is exquisitely specific of the antigen initially ingested or inhaled, and thus does not influence the development of systemic immune responses against other antigens, its manipulation has become an increasingly attractive strategy for preventing and possibly treating illnesses associated or resulting from the development of adverse immunological reactions against self and non-self antigens.

Mucosal tolerance and immunotherapy

Orally induced systemic tolerance had earlier been proposed as a strategy to prevent or to reduce the intensity of allergic reactions to chemical drugs [7, 12]. Later, the same rationale was followed in attempts to prevent or treat allergic reactions to common allergens [13-15]. More recently, nasal administration of a synthetic peptide (Der P1) entailing a dominant T cell epitope of house dust mite allergen could inhibit T cell and reaginic antibody responses in mice [16].

The phenomenon of mucosally induced systemic tolerance has likewise been utilized to reduce or suppress immune responses not only against foreign antigens but also against self antigens, *i.e.* components derived from host tissues. It has thus been possible to delay the onset and/or to decrease the intensity of experimental autoimmune diseases in a variety of animal systems by mucosal deposition of auto-antigens onto the intestinal (by feeding) or the respiratory mucosa (by aerosolization or intranasal instillation of antigens) [9]. For instance, oral administration of collagen type II has been shown to delay the onset of autoimmune arthritis in several animal models. Similarly, it has been possible to suppress an experimental form of autoimmune uveoretinitis by oral administration of the retinal S-antigen. Experimental autoimmune encephalomyelitis, a chronic relapsing demyelinating disorder that can be induced in susceptile strains of rodents by injection of purified myelin autoantigens or crude spinal cord homogenate together with adjuvant, can be suppressed partially or completely in animals fed myelin antigens or synthetic peptides thereof [9].

Although the above examples indicate that mucosal administration of foreign as well as self antigens offers good promise for inducing specific immunologic tolerance, the applicability of this approach in human and in veterinary medicine remains limited by practical problems. Indeed, to be clinically broadly applicable, mucosally-induced immunological tolerance must also be effective in patients in whom the disease process has already established itself and/or in whom potentially tissue-damaging immune cells already exist. This is especially important when considering strategies of tolerance induction in patients suffering from or prone to an autoimmune disease, an allergic condition, or a chronic inflammatory reaction to a persistent microorganism. Current protocols of mucosally induced tolerance have had limited success in suppressing the expression of an already established state of systemic immunological sensitization [17, 18]. This may partly explain the disappointing results of recent clinical trials of oral tolerance in patients with multiple sclerosis and rheumatoid arthritis [9].

In addition, and by analogy with mucosal vaccines aimed at inducing immune responses to infectious pathogens, induction of immunological tolerance by mucosal application of most antigens requires administration of massive amounts of antigens or prolonged administration of relatively smaller amounts of antigens which are then only effective in rather narrow dose ranges. A likely explanation is that most antigens are extensively degraded before entering a mucosal tissue and/or are absorbed in insufficient quantities.

Cholera toxin B subunit as mucosal carrier-immunomodulating system for antipathological vaccination

It has been widely assumed that strong mucosal immunogens such as protease-resistant molecules with mucosa-binding properties characteristically induce local and systemic immune responses when administered by the oral route without inducing immunological tolerance. Based on this assumption, mucosal administration of antigens coupled to mucosa-binding molecules such as CT or its mucosa-binding fragment CTB, has been proposed as a strategy to induce local and systemic immune responses rather than tolerance [19, 20]. Indeed some years ago, CT and CTB attracted interest not only as potent mucosal immunogens and carrier molecules for oral delivery of foreign protein antigens, but also as agents capable to abrogate systemic immunological tolerance when co-administered with various antigens/tolerogens [21].

In the course of recent studies, we have observed that physical coupling of an antigen to CTB led to alterations that resulted in hitherto unexpected effects: when given by various mucosal (oral, intranasal, vaginal, rectal) routes, CTB induced a strong mucosal IgA immune response to itself and in some cases also to the conjugated antigen, but instead of abrogating systemic tolerance to itself and to the conjugated antigens enhanced it profoundly [22].

Based on this unexpected finding and on the results of other experiments with a variety of soluble protein antigens and particulate antigens (reviewed in [23], we had good reasons to believe that such a system may be advantageous for inducing peripheral tolerance. First, it minimizes by several hundred-fold the amount of antigen/tolerogen and drastically reduces the number of doses that would otherwise be required by reported protocols of orally-induced tolerization. Second, but probably most important, this strategy appears to be applicable for preventing expression of an already established state of systemic immune sensitization. In the foregoing, we shall summarize the results of recent studies using this type of approach as a means to prevent or treat pathological immune responses associated with experimental autoimmune diseases, type I allergies, and allograft rejection.

Treatment of organ-specific autoimmune diseases: we have demonstrated that mucosal administration of relevant autoantigens linked to CTB could inhibit the development of clinical disease in animal models of experimentally inducible autoimmune diseases, such as allergic encephalomyelitis [24] and collagen-induced arthritis

[25]. In the latter system, nasal administration of a collagen type II-CTB conjugate could inhibit disease progression even when treatment was initiated after onset of clinically overt disease. Furthermore, oral treatment of female NOD mice with a CTB-insulin conjugate could suppress type I diabetes [26], a model of spontaneous autoimmune disease, even when given as late as 15 weeks post-birth (that is at a time when all mice have evidence of insulitis). In all of the models tested, protection against clinical disease was consistently associated with decreased IL-2 responses in lymph nodes draining the site of disease induction [22-25]. However, and depending on the nature of the conjugated antigen, the route of administration (oral, nasal) of the conjugate, and the animal species used, this type of treatment variably affected the capacity of lymph node T cells to produce stereotype Th1 (IFN-γ) or Th2 (IL-4, IL-5) cytokines upon *in vitro* re-exposure to the fed or inhaled autoantigen.

The most striking observation in all three models of autoimmune diseases tested was the finding that treatment with CTB-antigen suppressed leukocyte infiltration into the target organ [22-26]. This observation suggests that the mechanisms governing induction of tolerance by feeding or inhaling CTB-linked antigens may involve modifications of the migratory behavior of inflammatory cells. Assuming that protective T cells induced by CTB-mediated mucosal delivery of autoantigens, unlike inflammatory T cells, do not migrate into the target tissue, they may still leave the mucosa and, via the blood, reach draining lymph nodes where they could interfere with the recruitment and migration of inflammatory leukocytes. Supporting this interpretation are the results of adoptive co-transfer experiments between congenic NOD mice. Thus, injection of irradiated male Thy 1.2 recipients with diabetogenic T cells from syngeneic female mice and T cells from congenic Thy 1.1 mice fed with CTB-insulin, demonstrated a selective recruitment of Thy 1.1 donor cells in the peripancreatic lymph nodes concommitant with reduced islet cell infiltration [26]. These results suggest that treatment with CTB-autoantigen induces the selective migration and retention of protective T cells into lymphoid tissues draining the site of organ injury. Conversely, and without arguing with the latter interpretation, treatment with CTB-antigen may also induce the migration of inflammatory T cells or their precursors from the periphery into mucosal effector tissues where they could be anergized, deleted or even ignored. Further studies on the expression of adhesion molecules on protective cells and on inflammatory cells could be valuable.

Recent studies have demonstrated that CTB itself, even when administered systemically, induces profound down-regulation of systemic immune responses to co-administered antigens [27]. Collectively, these observations indicate that CTB not only acts as a powerful carrier delivery system to facilitate mucosal uptake of co-administered antigens but is also endowed with strong immunomodulating properties. Hence, this strategy of tolerance induction appears to involve mechanisms that are distinct from those governing induction of tolerance after mucosal administration of free antigens.

Prevention of graft rejection: by coupling thymocytes to cholera B subunit and feeding this conjugate to mice, we have also been able to significantly prolong the survival of transplanted hearts in allogeneic mouse recipients. (Sun, Czerkinsky and Holmgren, in preparation.) Recently, feeding CTB-derivatized donor keratinocytes has been shown to prevent corneal allograft rejection in mice (Niederkorn JR, personal communication).

Prevention of type I allergies: nasal administration of a soluble protein allergen (ovalbumin) linked to Escherichia coli heat-labile enterotoxin B subunit, a GM1-binding analogue of CTB, has been found to suppress systemic delayed hypersensitivity responses and IgE antibody responses in mice [28]. This observation is consistent with the recent finding that interferon-γ, IL-4 and IL-6 responses are decreased together with IgG1 and IgG2a antibody responses in animals given a nasal CTB-type II collagen vaccine [25], and indicates that, under certain conditions, this form of tolerance can affect both TH1- and TH2-driven responses.

Mucosal vaccine formulations for simultaneous induction of anti-infectious and anti-pathological immunity: the cholera toxin B subunit paradygm

Somewhat surprisingly, vaccinologists in general and mucosal immunologists in particular have usually believed a reciprocal relationship to exist between induction of immunity and tolerance. The observation that mucosal immunity, which is typified by secretory IgA antibodies, may develop concomitantly with systemic immunological tolerance [11], has led to the belief that vaccines against mucosal pathogens should primarily stimulate immunity without inducing tolerance. However, from a theoretical standpoint, the possibility to manipulate the mucosal immune system towards both immunity and tolerance appears rather attractive when considering strategies aimed at protecting the host from colonization or invasion by mucosal pathogens but also to interfere with the development of potentially harmful systemic immunological reactions against the same pathogens or their products.

The notion that peripheral T cell tolerance may be an efficient mechanism to protect against immunopathological reactions associated with certain infections has been illustrated by recent studies in mice. Whereas mice from a susceptible (BALB/c) background develop an early Th2-driven IL-4 response and ultimately succomb to their infection with *Leishmania major*, mice from the same background but rendered tolerant in the periphery after nasal administration of as little as 12 micrograms of *L. major* LACK antigen conjugated to CTB showed markedly delayed disease onset [29]. Such treatment was associated with decreased proliferative responses to LACK. An examination of cytokine responsiveness to LACK after mucosal tolerization with CTB-LACK revealed that while the Th1 response to LACK was suppressed, TH2 cytokine production (in terms of IL-4 and IL-5) was apparently unaffected. Most importantly, treatment with CTB-LACK reduced by almost 3 logs parasite burden in the skin and draining lymph nodes of infected mice [29].

Similar findings have also been observed in mice infested with the parasite nematode, *Schistosoma mansoni* (Sun *et al.*, in preparation). Thus, nasal treatment of mice with *S. mansoni* glutathione S transferase (GST) conjugated to CTB suppressed granuloma formation and decreased parasite burden and egg deposition in the liver of infested animals [30]. Protection with this nasal CTB-GST vaccine was associated with decreased systemic T cell proliferative responses to GST and reduced spontaneous proliferation of liver leukocytes. Hepatic production of IFN-γ, IL-5 and IL-3 were markedly reduced whereas that of IL-4 remained unaffected. Most importantly, such treatment could significantly prolong the survival of animals, even when initiated as late as 6 weeks after initial infection, that is at a time when liver granulomatous reactions are most pronounced.

These results lend promise for the development of a novel class of therapeutic vaccines against diseases associated with inflammatory reactions caused by persistent microorganisms and their products.

Conclusions and prospects

Such features should bear on the design of vaccines aimed at promoting SIgA immune responses against the numerous infectious pathogens that enter the host through mucosal membranes, and at protecting the host from developing potentially harmful cell-mediated immune responses against the same matters. The relative inefficiency of injectable vaccines to evoke secretory IgA immune responses in mucosal tissues and the fact that they can induce DTH reactivity and thereby bystander tissue damage upon subsequent encounter with the corresponding pathogen constitute two major reasons to encourage the development of alternative strategies to stimulate appropriate immune responses in MALT. Mucosal administration of antigens may theoretically result in the concomitant expression of SIgA antibody responses in various mucosal tissues and secretions, and under appropriate conditions, in the simultanous down-regulation of cell-mediated immune reactivity at local and systemic sites. Thus, developing formulations based on efficient delivery of selected antigens/tolerogens, cytokines and adjuvants may impact on the design of future vaccines and of specific immunotherapeutic agents to prevent and/or treat diseases or conditions associated with untoward tissue-damaging immune responses, such as certain autoimmune diseases and allograft rejection.

Acknowledgements

The studies summarized here were supported in part by the European Communities (Biotech Programme), the Swedish Medical Research Council, the Institut National de la Santé et de la Recherche Médicale (France), and Triotol (Sweden).

References

1. Brandtzaeg P. Basic mechanisms of mucosal immunity: a major adaptive defence system. *The Immunologist* 1995; 3: 89-95.
2. Guy-Grand D, Griscelli DC, Vassali P. The mouse gut lymphocyte: a novel type of T cell: nature, origin, and traffic in mice in normal and graft-*versus*-host conditiond. *J Exp Med* 1978, 148, 1661-71.
3. Tagliabue A, Luini W, Doldateschi D, Botaschi D. Natural killer activity of gut mucosal lymphoid cells in mice. *Eur J Immunol* 1981, 11: 919-22.
4. MacDermott RP, Franklin GO, Jenkins RM, Kodner IJ, Nash GS, Weinrieb IJ. Human intestinal mononuclear cells. I. Investigation of antibody-dependent, lectin-induced and spontaneous cell-mediated cytotoxic capabilities. *Gastroenterology* 1980, 78: 47-56.
5. McGhee JR, Mestecky J. Mucosal vaccines: areas arising. In Kyiono H, Ernst P, eds. *Mucosal immunology update.* New York: Raven Press, 1993 (vol. 4): 1-19.
6. Holmgren, J, Lycke, N, Czerkinsky, C. Cholera toxin and cholera B subunit as oral-mucosal adjuvant and antigen vector systems. *Vaccine* 1993; 11: 1179-84.
7. Wells H. Studies on the chemistry of anaphylaxis III. Experiments with isolated proteins, especially those of hen's egg. *J Infect Dis* 1911; 9: 147-71.
8. Mowat AM. The regulation of immune responses to dietary protein antigens. *Immunol Today* 1987; 8: 93-8.
9. Weiner HL. Oral tolerance: immune mechanisms and treatment of autoimmune diseases. *Immunol Today* 1997; 18: 335-43.
10. Czerkinsky C, Holmgren J. The mucosal immune system: Anti-infectious and anti-inflammatory properties. *The Immunologist* 1995; 3: 97-103.
11. Challacombe SJ, Tomasi TB Jr. Systemic tolerance and secretory immunity after oral immunization. *J Exp Med* 1980; 152: 1459-72.
12. Chase MW. Inhibition of experimental drug allergy by prior feeding of the sensitizing agent. *Proc Soc Exp Biol* 1946; 61: 257-9.
13. Wortmann F. Oral hyposensitization of children with pollinosis or house dust asthma. *Allergol Immunopathol* 1977; 5: 15-26.
14. Rebien W, Puttonen E, Maasch HJ, Stix E, Wahn U. Clinical and immunological response to oral and subcutaneous immunotherapy with grass pollen extracts. A prospective study. *Eur J Pediatry* 1982; 138: 341-4.
15. Holt PG. Immunoprophylaxis of atopy: light at the end of the tunnel? *Immunol Today* 1994; 15: 484-9.
16. Hoyne GF, O'Hehir RE, DC Wraith, Thomas WR, Lamb JR. Inhibition of T cell and antibody responses to house dust mite allergen by inhalation of the dominant T cell epitope in naïve and sensitized mice. *J Exp Med* 1993; 178: 1783-8.
17. Hansson DG, Vaz NM, Rawlings LA, Lynch JM. Inhibition of specific immune responses by feeding protein antigens. II. Effects of prior passive and active immunization. *J Immunol* 1979; 122: 2261-6.
18. Staines NA, Harper N, Ward FJ, Thompson HSG, Bansal S. Arthritis: animal models of oral tolerance. *Ann NY Acad Sci* 1996; 778: 297-305.
19. McKenzie SJ, Halsey JF. Cholera toxin B subunit as a carrier protein to stimulate a mucosal immune response. *J Immunol* 1984; 133: 1818-24.
20. De Aizpurua HJ, Russell-Jones GJ. Oral vaccination. Identification of classes of proteins that provoke an immune response upon oral feeding. *J Exp Med* 1988; 167: 440-51.
21. Elson CO, Ealding W. Cholera toxin did not induce oral tolerance in mice and abrogated oral tolerance to an unrelated antigen. *J Immunol* 1984; 133: 2892-8.

22. Sun JB, Holmgren J, Czerkinsky C. Cholera toxin B subunit: an effective tansmucosal carrier delivery system for induction of peripheral immunological tolerance. *Proc Natl Acad Sci USA* 1994; 91: 10795-9.
23. Czerkinsky C, Sun JB, Lebens M, Li BL, Rask C, Lindblad M, Holmgren J. Cholera toxin B subunit as transmucosal carrier-delivery and immunomodulating system for induction of anti-infectious and anti-pathological immunity. *Ann NY Acad Sci* 1996; 778: 185-93.
24. Sun, JB, Rask C, Olsson T, Holmgren J, Czerkinsky C. Treatment of experimental autoimmune encephalomyelitis by feeding myelin basic protein conjugated to cholera toxin B subunit. *Proc Natl Acad Sci USA* 1996; 93: 7196-201.
25. Tarkowski A, Sun JB, Holmdal R, Holmgren J, Czerkinsky C. Treatment of experimental autoimmune arthritis by nasal administration of a type II collagen-cholera B subunit conjugate vaccine, 1998 submitted.
26. Bergerot I, Ploix C, Petersen J, Moulin V, Rask C, Fabien N, Lindblad M, Mayer A, Czerkinsky C, Holmgren J, Thivolet C. A cholera toxoid-insulin conjugate as oral vaccine against spontaneous autoimmune diabetes. *Proc Natl Acad Sci USA* 1997; 94: 4610-4.
27. Williams NA, Stasiuk LM, Nashar TO, Richards CM, Lang AK, Day MJ, Hirst TR. Prevention of autoimmune disease due to lymphocyte modulation by the B-subunit of *Escherichia coli* heat-labile enterotoxin. *Proc Natl Acad Sci USA* 1997; 94: 5290-5.
28. Tamura S, Hatori E, Tsuruhara T, Aizawa C, Kurata T. Suppression of delayed-type hypersensitivity and IgE antibody responses to ovalbumin by intranasal administration of *Escherichia coli* heat-labile enterotoxin B subunit-conjugated ovalbumin. *Vaccine* 1997; 15: 225-9.
29. Mc Sorley SJ, Rask C, Pichot R, Julia V, Czerkinsky C, Glaichenhaus N. Selective tolerization of Th1-like cells after nasal administration of a cholera toxoid-LACK conjugate. *Eur J Immunol* 1998; 28: in press.
30. Sun JB, Mielcarek N., Lakew M, Grzych JM, Capron A, Holmgren J, Czerkinsky C. Intranasal administration of a schistosoma mansoni glutathione-S-transferase-cholera toxoid conjugate vaccine evokes anti-parasite and anti-pathological immunity in mice, submitted, 1998.

Recent advances in the pathogenesis of gastrointestinal bacterial infections.
P. Rampal, P. Boquet, eds. John Libbey Eurotext, Paris © 1998, pp. 165-174.

Immunomodulatory properties of cholera toxin and related enterotoxins

Timothy R. Hirst, Toufic O. Nashar, Douglas G. Millar, Neil A. Williams

Department of Pathology and Microbiology, School of Medical Sciences, University of Bristol, Bristol BS8 1TD, UK

Cholera-toxin (Ctx) from *Vibrio cholerae* and the related heat-labile enterotoxin (Etx) from *Escherichia coli* are now recognised as having remarkable immunological properties, in addition to their established roles as mediators of diarrhoeal disease. The toxins trigger extremely potent anti-toxin antibody responses following systemic immunisation, even when administered in the absence of a conventional adjuvant; and they also elicit vigorous mucosal responses, which makes them almost unique among soluble proteins. These findings are interesting in their own right, but studies have also shown that the toxins can act as adjuvants, stimulating either systemic or mucosal responses to other co-administered or conjugated antigens. This has resulted in the inclusion of Ctx or Etx in putative mucosal vaccines against infectious diseases. However, concerns over the inherent toxicity of Ctx and Etx have led to attempts to separate their toxic and adjuvant properties by creating either non-toxic variants or by using components of the toxins devoid of diarrhoeagenic activity. The toxins are comprised of a single A-subunit in association with five B-subunits. Studies have shown that mutations which ablate the ADP-ribosyltransferase activity of the A-subunit, give rise to holotoxins which retain adjuvant properties. Recombinant preparations of B-subunits, completely devoid of any toxicity, have also been found to retain significant adjuvant activity. However, somewhat paradoxically, the B-subunits of Ctx and Etx also promote tolerance to autoantigens, which has important implications for their use in preventing inflammatory autoimmune diseases. These toxins can therefore be considered as potent immunomodulators, which function by interacting in a complex fashion with the immune system. By understanding the structural and functional properties responsible for their inherent immunogenicity and striking adjuvant and toleragenic activities, it should be possibl to rationally exploit these molecules as immunostimulatory components of vaccines and as therapeutic agents for the prevention of autoimmune disease.

Toxin structure and mode of action

Ctx and Etx are comprised of an A-subunit with ADP-ribosyltransferase activity and five B-subunits which bind to a ubiquitous glycosphingolipid, GM1 ganglioside [Gal(β1-3)GalNAc(β1-4){NeuAc(α2-3)}Gal(β1-4)Glc(β1-1)ceramide], found on the surfaces of eukaryotic cells [1, 2]. The similarity in structure and function between the two toxins stems from their high degree of sequence identity (82% at the amino acid level) [3]. The A-subunit (CtxA and EtxA) can be readily nicked by exogenous proteases to yield two fragments, A_1 (with ADP-ribosylating activity) and A_2, linked to one another by a disulphide bridge [4]. The enterotoxic activity of Ctx and Etx is attributable to the A_1-fragment which enters the cell cytosol and triggers Cl^- efflux by catalysing ADP-ribosylation of Gsa which in turn activates adenylate cyclase and leads to a concomitant elevation in cAMP levels. Raised cAMP causes protein kinase A to phosphorylate and open the cystic fibrosis transmembrane conductance (CFTR) Cl^- channel. Cl^- efflux results in the osmotic movement of water from enterocytes into the gut lumen, giving rise to profuse watery diarrhoea characteristic of cholera and related enteropathies. The A_2-fragment represents an adapter responsible for interaction with the B-subunit pentamer [1]. The C-terminus of the A_2-fragment, which emerges on the opposite face of the B pentamer from the A_1-fragment contains a -KDEL sequence motif (-RDEL in Etx) normally involved in the retrieval of proteins from the trans-Golgi network (TGN) to the endoplasmic reticulum (ER) [5]. The -KDEL sequence has been found to contribute to the efficiency of toxin action [6], and may also play a role in modulating the immunological effects of the toxins (see below).

The B-subunits of Ctx and Etx (CtxB and EtxB, respectively) are assembled into a doughnut-shaped pentameric ring. The interactions between adjacent B-subunit monomers in the pentamer involve three-stranded anti-parallel β-sheets (on each adjacent subunit) as well as a high number of salt-bridges, making the B pentamer one of the most stable non-covalently associated subunit complexes known [7]. In this regard, the B-subunits are stable in conditions that normally lead to protein degradation or denaturation, with the molecule remaining pentameric in 1 mg/ml trypsin or proteinase K, at acid pH's as low as 2.0, in 8.0 M urea and ionic detergents such as sodium dodecyl sulphate. The function of EtxB and CtxB is to mediate interaction with cell surface receptors which permits toxin internalisation and the delivery of the A-subunit into the cell. CtxB and EtxB interact with the pentasaccharide moiety of GM1-ganglioside [8-10]. This results in high affinity binding with reported dissociation constants for interaction with GM1 of 7.3×10^{-10} M for CtxB and 5.7×10^{-10} M for EtxB [11]. Athough the main receptor fro EtxB and CtxB is GM1, the subunits also show some affinity for GD1b, but the dissociation constants are approximately one order of magnitude lower than those for GM1. In addition, EtxB has been reported to interact with other cell surface receptors, notably asialo-GM1, lactosylceramide, and certain galactoproteins [12-15]. The consequence of these differential binding specificities on the biological and immunological properties of Ctx and Etx have yet to be fully evaluated, thus caution is needed in assuming that observations on EtxB will be identical to those of CtxB.

Why are cholera toxin and related enterotoxins such potent immunogens?

By contrast to most soluble proteins Ctx and Etx are exceptionally potent immunogens. Normally, the parenteral immunisation of a protein leads to low level antibody responses unless it is administered in combination with a suitable adjuvant, such as Freund's adjuvant or Alum. However, Ctx and Etx induce high level antibody responses even when injected in normal saline or water. In addition, if Ctx or Etx are administered to mucosal sites they induce strong local IgA and systemic antibody production [16, 17], whereas conventional soluble antigens usually either fail to trigger an immune response or induce specific tolerance.

Immunisation of mice or rabbits with Ctx or Etx results in high titre antibody responses directed against the B-subunit component of the toxin, suggesting that the B-subunit is immunodominant. When congenic strains of mice were orally immunised with recombinant preparations of the B-subunits of Ctx or Etx it was found that the magnitude of serum anti-B-subunit responses were H-2 linked. For example, mice of the H-2^b haplotype (B10 or C57/BL/6) responded exceptionally well to CtxB, whereas H-2^d mice (B10.D2 or BALB/c) proved to be high responders to EtxB, but relatively low responders to CtxB [18]. These observations are consistent with the recent identification of different immunodominant T-cell epitopes in CtxB (residues 89-100) and EtxB (residues 36-44), respectively [19, 20].

In our laboratory we have sought to identify the functional attributes of the B-subunits responsible for their exceptionally potent immunogenicity. Since the B-subunit's primary function is to bind to cell surfaces, we used site-directed mutagenesis to generate a mutant EtxB subunit containing a glycine to aspartate substitution at residue 33 so as to inhibit receptor-recognition [17]. The resultant mutant, EtxB(G33D) forms indistinguishable pentameric complexes to wild-type B-subunit, as revealed by X-ray crystallography, and retains all of its physicochemical properties, except the ability to bind to GM1 ganglioside receptors [17, 21]. A comparison of the antibody responses elicited by EtxB and EtxB(G33D) demonstrated that the potent immunogenicity of the B-subunit is fully dependent on receptor recognition [17]. Mice immunised subcutaneously (s.c.) or orally with EtxB produced high titre antibody responses to the B-subunit, whereas those given EtxB(G33D) produced only meagre responses following s.c. injection, and failed to elicit any response after oral immunisation.

An analysis of *in vitro* lymph node responses from mice immunised with EtxB revealed that addition of wild-type EtxB strikingly altered the distribution of lymphocyte subsets compared to those found in the presence of EtxB(G33D). Notably, by day 4 of culture EtxB had caused an increase in the proportion of B-cells, many of which were activated, as evidenced by the upregulation of the low-affinity IL-2 receptor (CD25) [17]. In addition, the presence of EtxB in such cultures triggered the complete depletion of $CD8^+$ T-cells [17]. A similar pattern of responses was observed when EtxB was added to cultures of mesenteric lymph node cells responding to an unrelated antigen, namely ovalbumin [22]. Subsequent studies revealed that addition of EtxB, but not EtxB(G33D), to lymphocyte cultures, triggered $CD8^+$

T-cells to undergo apoptosis [22]. This occurred over a period of 12-16 h and explains the observed depletion of this population of T-cells from lymph node cells cultured in the presence of EtxB. A similar effect may also occur *in vivo*; since oral administration of CtxB causes a reduction in $CD8^+$ T-cells from both the Peyer's patch and intraepithelial lymphocyte (IEL) compartments [23]. It is, however, not yet clear what effects depletion of this subset of cells would have on the outcome of the immune response to EtxB or CtxB *in vivo*. $CD8^+$ T-cells are associated with a regulatory role in the immune response, arising from production of specific cytokines such as interferon-γ (IFNγ). The loss of immunoregulation by this cytokine should favour induction of T-helper 2 (Th2) T-cell responses, characterised by the production of IL-4, IL-5, and IL-10, and induction of high levels of antibodies of the IgG1 and IgE classes, as well as suppression of cell-mediated immunity. Consistent with this is the observation that the IgG1 subclass predominates following immunisation with EtxB, and that EtxB induces a Th2-dominated response to cadministered antigens (see below).

The effect of EtxB and CtxB on B-cells and $CD4^+$ T-cells has also been investigated. Incubation of EtxB with lymphocyte cultures, depleted of adherent cells, caused the generalised activation of naive B-cells with upregulation of surface markers such as MHC Class II, B7, CD25, CD40 and ICAM-1 [24]. This occurred in the absence of significant proliferation in cultures containing both B- and T-cells, indicating that EtxBdoes not have a mitogenic activity. Further investigations using highly purified B-cells, revealed that EtxB caused upregulated expression of MHC Class II and CD25, implying that the effect on other surface markers was likely to be the consequence of increased interaction with $CD4^+$ T-cells present in the original cultures (Nashar – unpublished observations). CtxB has also been shown to elevate the expression of MHC Class II on naive B-cells [25]. Preliminary studies have also revealed that EtxB-receptor binding triggers upregulation of several adhesion and costimulatory molecules on $CD4^+$ T-cells, and may trigger secretion of Th2-associated cytokines (Nashar, Lang, Hirst & Williams – unpublished observations). While the degree of surface expression of MHC molecules, co-stimulatory and adhesion proteins, and secreted cytokines may ultimately enhance or modulate the T-cell response to presented antigens, productive processing of the protein and loading of antigenic epitopes onto MHC class II molecules is essential for T-cell receptor (TcR) signalling.

Normally, antigen presenting cells (APCs) such as dendritic cells, macrophages, B-cells, and intestinal epithelial cells internalise foreign antigen by macropinocytosis, phagocytosis, and receptor-mediated endocytosis (for a review see [26]). This results in the antigen being taken into endosomes and subsequently trafficked through intracellular compartments of distinct composition and pH. The early endosomes are progressively acidified and mature into late endosomes that fuse with lysosomes where their contents are proteolytically digested. The activity of proteases at various stages in the pathway can generate peptides fragments containing antigenic epitopes. Newly synthesised MHC class II molecules, in association with invariant-chain protein (Ii) are transported *via* a secretory pathway that intersects with the endocytic pathway containing processed antigen. The peptide epitope is loaded onto the class II molecule, Ii is removed, and the assembled complex is routed to the cell surface. The uptake, processing and presentation of toxin-derived epitopes by APCs remains to be fully evaluated. It is however conceivable that the ability of the B-subunits to bind to GM1, trigger uptake and sequester endosomal trafficking pathways might influence the generation of toxin derived epitopes and their loading onto class II. This may be most relevant in relation to the APC function of B cells where levels of antigen uptake, other than specific uptake through surface membrane immunoglobulin is normally low. Thus the GM1-mediated uptake of B-subunits might allow non-toxin specific B-cells to function as APCs in the presentation of toxin derived epitopes. In addition, toxins might alter intracellular trafficking pathways, causing the re-routing of antigen to intracellular compartments containing different proteolytic enzymes, and thereby altering peptide epitope liberation and destruction, and possibly improving peptide loading onto MHC class II. Somewhat paradoxically, Harding and coworkers recently demonstrated hat pre-treatment of Listeria-elicited peritoneal macrophages with cholera toxin inhibited the processing and presentation of hen egg lysozyme (HEL) to a HEL epitope-specific T-cell hybridoma [27]. Similar inhibition of antigen processing by *E. coli* enterotoxin was also found [28]. Work in our laboratory has shown that treatment of the macrophage cell line, J774, with recombinant EtxB also inhibits the processing and presentation of heterologous antigens such as ovalbumin and HEL to T-cell specific hybridomas (Millar & Hirst, unpublished observations). Intriguingly, the J774 cells become highly vacuolated, suggesting that EtxB induces an alteration in the sorting and trafficking of intracellular membranes. This finding is reminiscent of the effect of a vacuolating toxin, VacA, from *Helicobacter pylori* which has been shown to decrease invariant chain-dependent antigen processing, MHC class II loading, and presentation of tetanus toxin (TT) by B-cells [29]. VacA induces acidic vacuoles containing late endosomal and lysosomal markers [30], perhaps sequestering the essential antigen processing machinery needed for efficient TT presentation.

How can inhibition of antigen processing be reconciled with the observed increase in immune responses generated by the enterotoxins? Sustained T-cell responses and memory responses may require antigen to persist, undegraded, for extended periods of time. Retention of antigen in mildly-acidic compartments has been observed in immature dendritic cells and it has been postulated that delayed processing may be important in allowing efficient antigen presentation to T-cells following migration to the lymph node [31].

It thus seems likely that the potent immunogenicity of Ctx, Etx and their respective B-subunits is due to a multitude of effects which can be chiefly attributed to the B-subunits ability to bind to cell-surface receptors, namely, i) improved uptake into APCs, ii) alterations in membrane trafficking leading to persistence and sustained presentation of the antigen, iii) the potential recruitment of B-cells into the process of antigen presentation, iv) the induced expression of costimulatory and adhesion molecules leading to enhanced cognate interaction between APCs and $CD4^+$ T-cells, and v) an alteration in the balance of cytokine secretion resulting in the differentiation of $CD4^+$ Th2 cells and their subsequent help in the expansion of toxin-specific B-cells secreting high levels of antibodies directed against the B-subunit.

Enterotoxins and their B-subunits as adjuvants and therapeutic agents

The discovery that Ctx could act as an adjuvant for antibody responses towards other antigens was first reported in 1972 [32]. It was subsequently shown that mucosal immune responses to a wide variety of soluble antigens could be induced if they were administered in combination with small quantities of Ctx [33]. This provided a unique opportunity to investigate the mucosal immune system and to develop effective mucosally delivered vaccines.

The explanation of why Ctx and Etx adjuvant responses to other antigens has been confounded by apparently conflicting observations on the importance and significance of the individual A- and B-subunits. For example, the analysis of a mutant of *E. coli* heat-labile enterotoxin, with a Glu to Lys substitution in residue 112 of the A-subunit, revealed that it was inactive both as a toxin and as an adjuvant [34]. This led to the conclusion that adjuvanticity and toxicity were inseparable, and that the adjuvanticity was dependent on the ADP-ribosylation function of the A-subunit. However, subsequent studies have provided definitive evidence that mutant toxins which render the molecules inactive in a wide range of *in vitro* and *in vivo* ADP-ribosylation assays, still function as adjuvants [35, 36]. In addition, it was observed that recombinant EtxB acted as a poor adjuvant, while CtxB lacked adjuvanticity altogether [35, 37]. This has led to the view that a combination of properties in the A-subunit (both enzymatic and non-enzymatic) and the delivery function of the B-subunits confer adjuvanticity to these toxins. The A-subunit contains important targeting signals such as a C-terminal -KDEL retention sequence and an ARF-binding site which might alter vesicular traffic and thereby enhance the targeting of coadministered antigens to compartments where improved processing and presentation can occur. However, it should be noted that there have been a number of reports which indicate that the B-subunits (devoid of any contaminating A-subunit) possess immunomodulatory properties [25, 38, 39]. For example, this laboratory has shown that an intranasal vaccine comprising a mixture of glycoproteins from herpes simplex virus (HSV), administered with recombinant EtxB as the adjuvant, afforded high level protection to ocular challenge with virulent HSV (Williams, Richards & Hill – unpublished observations). Thus, the B-subunits of Etx and Ctx should not be considered solely as delivery vehicles for their resective A-subunits, but as potentiators of immune responses in their own right. This should not be surprising given the profound effects of the B-subunits on leukocyte populations (see above). Therefore, Ctx and Etx should be considered as composite molecules, in which B-subunit receptor-interaction activates signalling pathways that activate APCs (and other immune cells) and influences antigen uptake, while the A-subunit further augments uptake and traffic of coadministered antigen into appropriate intracellular compartments and also elevates cAMP that alters gene expression and cell activation. Not too surprisingly, therefore, the fully active holotoxin remains the best adjuvant, although because of its inherent toxicity it is unlikely to find use as a component of human vaccines. By contrast, the non-toxic derivatives of Etx, as well as EtxB are emerging as safe, credible alternatives.

In light of the above discussion, it is important to note that CtxB and EtxB have recently been shown to potentiate immunological tolerance, which is somewhat of a paradox given their evident adjuvant properties. Czerkinsky, Holmgren *et al.* have coupled various antigens to CtxB, and shown that the oral administration of the conjugates induces peripheral tolerance to the attached antigen [40-42]. Their initial studies, based on the coupling of sheep red blood cells and bovine gamma globulin to CtxB, have now been extended to myelin basic protein (MBP) and insulin and shown to effectively suppress systemic T cell reactivity in experimental allergic encephalomyelitis (EAE) in the rat and diabetes in the NOD mouse, respectively [41-43]. In addition, we have reported that EtxB (but not EtxB(G33D) can completely prevent the induction of collagen induced arthritis (CIA) in DBA/1 mice when given subcutaneously at the same time as injection with collagen [39]. The fact that EtxB used in these experiments was administered *via* a non-mucosal route, indicates that the toleragenic activity of the B-subunit is not due to induction of oral tolerance in a conventional sense, but rather to a modulation of the immune response to the autoantigen. In this respect, the protection from induction of arthritis by EtxB was found to coincide with a shift in the nature of the immune response to collagen, away from a Th1-dominated response to one favouring Th2 activation, characterised by high levels of IL-4 secretion and increased relative IgG1 production [39]. Thus, EtxB and CtxB can be considered as agents which modulate the nature of T-helper cell differentiation and/or activity by suppressing pro-inflammatory Th1 responses and stimulating Th2 responses. This also explains why the B-subunit can be both a putative adjuvant and a toleragen, since in both circumstances a shift towards a Th2 response will be beneficial. In the case of vaccines, in which B-subunits are incorporated as adjuvants, a Th2 response should increas the level of antigen-specific secretory IgA and serum IgG production, thereby affording greater protection against infectious agents and virulence determinants. Whereas, an EtxB-mediated Th2 response to autoantigens should deviate the immune system away from inflammatory responses that normally lead to tissue damage and disease. This heralds the possibility that EtxB and CtxB will find therapeutic applications in controlling a range of inflammatory disorders, including multiple sclerosis, type I diabetes, and autoimmune uveitis. All of these diseases are thought to be initiated by autoreactive Th1 cells [44], and evidence from relevant experimental models suggests that protection can be afforded by the induction of a Th2 response.

Concluding remarks

The recent advances in our understanding of the mechanisms of activity of cholera toxin and related enterotoxins have clearly opened up new possibilities for their use as adjuvants and immunotherapeutic agents. Thus, bacterial toxins which have wrought havoc as agents of diarrhoeal diseases, are set to make an enormous beneficial impact on human medicine.

Acknowledgements

We would wish to thank The Wellcome Trust, the Arthritis and Rheumatism Council and the Medical Research Councils of Great Britain and Canada for their generous financial support. T.O.N. and D.G.M. are recipients of a Wellcome Trust Research Fellowship and Canadian MRC Fellowship, respectively.

References

1. Sixma T, Kalk K, van Zanten B, Dauter Z, Kingma J, Witholt B, Hol W. Refined structure of *Escherichia coli* heat-labile enterotoxin, a close relative of cholera toxin. *J Mol Biol* 1993; 230: 890-918.
2. Merritt EA, Sarfaty S, Akker F, L'hoir C, Martial J, Hol WGJ. Crystal structure of cholera toxin B-pentamer bound to receptor GM1 pentasaccharide. *Prot Sci* 1994; 3: 166-75.
3. Domenighini M, Pizza M, Jobling MG, Holmes RK, Rappuoli R. Identification of errors among database sequence entries and comparison of correct amino acid sequences for the heat-labile enterotoxins of *Escherichia coli* and *Vibrio cholerae*. *Mol Microbiol* 1995; 15: 1165-7.
4. Merritt EA, Pronk SE, Sixma TK, Kalk KH, Vanzanten BAM, Hol WGJ. Structure of partially-activated *Escherichia coli* heat-labile enterotoxin (LT) at 2.6-A resolution. *FEBS Letters* 1994; 337: 88-92.
5. Pelham HRB. The Florey lecture, 1992: the secretion of proteins by cells. *Proc Royal Soc London, Series B* 1992; 250: 1-10.
6. Lencer WI, Constable C, Moe S, Jobling MG, Webb HM, Ruston S, Madara JL, Hirst TR, Holmes RK. Targeting of cholera toxin and *Escherichia coli* heat-labile toxin in polarized epithelia – role of COOH-terminal KDEL. *J Cell Biol* 1995; 131: 951-62.
7. Ruddock LW, Ruston SP, Kelly SM, Price NC, Freedman RB, Hirst TR. Kinetics of acid-mediated disassembly of the B-subunit pentamer of *Escherichia coli* heat-labile enterotoxin – molecular basis of pH stability. *J Biol Chem* 1995; 270: 29953-8.
8. Cuatrecasas. Gangliosides and membrane receptors for cholera toxin. *Biochemistry* 1973; 12: 3558-66.
9. Holmgren J. Comparison of the tissue receptors for *Vibrio cholerae* and *Escherichia coli* enterotoxins by means of gangliosides and natural cholera toxoid. *Infect Immun* 1973; 8: 851-9.
10. Van Heyningen WE, Carpenter CCJ, Pierce NF, Greenough BI. Deactivation of cholera toxin by ganglioside. *J Infect Dis* 1971; 124: 415-8.
11. Kuziemko GM, Stroh M, Stevens RC. Cholera toxin binding and specificity for gangliosides determined by surface plasmon resonance. *Biochemistry* 1996; 35: 6375-84.
12. Bäckström M, Shahabi V, Johansson S, Teneberg S, Kjellberg A, Miller-Podrazo H, Holmgren J, Lebens J. Structural basis for differential receptor binding of cholera toxin and *Escherichia coli* heat-labile toxins: influence of heterologous amino acid substitutions in the cholera B-subunit. *Mol Microbiol* 1997; 24: 489-98.
13. Orlandi PA, Critchley DR, Fishman PH. The heat-labile enterotoxin of *Escherichia coli* binds to polylactosaminoglycan-containing receptors in Caco-2 human intestinal epithelial cells. *Biochemistry* 1994; 33: 12886-95.

14. Karlsson KA, Teneberg S, Angstrom J, Kjellberg A, Hirst TR, Bergstrom J, Miller Podraza H. Unexpected carbohydrate cross-binding by *Escherichia coli* heat-labile enterotoxin. Recognition of human and rabbit target cell glycoconjugates in comparison with cholera toxin. *Bioorganic Med Chem* 1996; 4: 1919-28.
15. Teneberg S, Hirst TR, Angstrom J, Karlsson KA. Comparison of the glycolipid-binding specificities of cholera toxin and porcine *Escherichia coli* heat-labile enterotoxin – identification of a receptor-active non-ganglioside glycolipid for the heat-labile toxin in infant rabbit small intestine. *Glycoconjugate J* 1994; 11: 533-40.
16. Nashar TO, Amin T, Marcello A, Hirst TR. Current progress in the development of the B subunits of cholera toxin and *Escherichia coli* heat-labile enterotoxin as carriers for the oral delivery of heterologous antigens and epitopes. *Vaccine* 1993; 11: 235-40.
17. Nashar TO, Webb HM, Eaglestone S, Williams NA, Hirst TR. Potent immunogenicity of the B-subunits of *E. coli* heat-labile enterotoxin: receptor binding is essential and induces differential modulation of lymphocyte subsets. *Proc Natl Acad Sci USA* 1996; 93: 226-30.
18. Nashar TO, Hirst TR. Immunoregulatory role of H-2 and Intra-H-2 alleles on antibody responses to recombinant preparations of B-subunits of *Escherichia coli* heat-labile enterotoxin (rEtxB) and cholera toxin (rCtxB). *Vaccine* 1995; 13: 803-10.
19. Cong YZ, Bowdon HR, Elson CO. Identification of immunodominant T-cell epitope on cholera toxin. *Eur J Immunol* 1996; 26: 2587-94.
20. Takahashi I, Kiyono H, Jackson RJ, Fujihashi K, Staats HF, Hamada S, Clements JD, Bost KL, McGhee JR. Epitope maps of the *Escherichia coli* heat-labile toxin B-subunit for development of synthetic oral vaccine. *Infect Immun* 1996; 64: 1290-8.
21. Merritt EA, Safaty S, Jobling MG, Holmes RK, Hirst TR, Hol WGJ. Structural studies of receptor binding by cholera toxin mutants. *Prot Sci* 1997; 6: 1516-28.
22. Nashar TO, Williams NA, Hirst TR. Cross-linking of cell-surface ganglioside GM1 induces the selective apoptosis of mature $CD8^+$ T-lymphocytes. *Int Immunol* 1996; 8: 731-6.
23. Elson CO, Holland SP, Dertzbaugh MT, Cuff CF, Anderson AO. Morphologic and functional alterations of mucosal T-cells by cholera toxin B-subunit. *J Immunol* 1995; 154: 1032-40.
24. Nashar TO, Hirst TR, Williams NA. Modulation of B-cell activation by the B-subunit of *Escherichia coli* heat-labile enterotoxin: receptor interaction upregulates MHC Class II, B7, CD40, CD25 and ICAM1. *Immunology* 1997; 91: 572-8.
25. Francis ML, Ryan J, Jobling MG, Holmes RK, Moss J, Mond JJ. Cyclic AMP-independent effects of cholera toxin on B-cell activation. 2. Binding of ganglioside-GM1 induces B-cell activation. *J Immunol* 1992; 148: 1999-2005.
26. Watts C. Capture and processing of exogenous antigens for presentation on MHC molecules. *Ann Rev Immunol* 1997; 15: 821-50.
27. Matousek MP, Nedrud JG, Harding CV. Distinct effects of recombinant cholera toxin B subunit and holotoxin on different stages of class II MHC antigen processing and presentation by macrophages. *J Immunol* 1996; 156: 4137-45.
28. Matousek MP, Nedrud JG, Cieplak W, Harding CV. *E. coli* heat labile enterotoxin and cholera toxin inhibit class II MHC antigen processing. *J Allergy Clin Immunol* 1997; 99: SS938.
29. Molinari M, Galli C, Norais N, Telford JL, Rappuoli R, Luzio JP, Montecucco C. Vacuoles induced by *Helicobacter pylori* toxin contain both late endosomal and lysosomal markers. *J Biol Chem* 1997; 272: 25339-44.
30. Molinari M, Salio M, Galli C, Norais N, Rappuoli R, Lanzavecchia A, Montecucco C. Selective inhibition of Ii-dependent antigen presentation by *Helicobacter pylori* toxin VacA. *J Exp Med* 1998; 187: 135-40.
31. Lutz MB, Rovere P, Kleijmeer MJ, Rescigno M, Assmann CU, Oorschot VMJ, Geuze HJ, Trucy J, Demandolx D, Davoust J, RicciardiCastagnoli P. Intracellular routes and selective

retention of antigens in mildly acidic cathepsin D/lysosome-associated membrane protein-1/MHC class II-positive vesicles in immature dendritic cells. *J Immunol* 1997; 159: 3707-16.
32. Northrup RS, Fauci AS. Adjuvant effect of cholera toxin on the immune response of the mouse to sheep red blood cells. *J Infect Dis* 1972; 125: 672-3.
33. Elson CO, Ealding W. Cholera toxin feeding did not induce oral tolerance in mice and abrogated oral tolerance to an unrelated antigen. *J Immunol* 1984; 133: 2892-7.
34. Lycke N, Tsuji T, Holmgren J. The adjuvant effect of *Vibrio cholerae* and *Escherichia coli* enterotoxins is linked to their ADP-ribosyl transferase activity. *Eur J Immunol* 1992; 22: 2277-81.
35. Douce G, Turcotte C, Cropley I, Roberts M, Pizza M, Domenghini M, Rappuoli R, Dougan G. Mutants in *Escherichia coli* heat-labile enterotoxin lacking ADP-ribosyltransferase activity act as non-toxic, mucosal adjuvants. *Proc Natl Acad Sci USA* 1995; 92: 1644-8.
36. De Haan L, Verweij WR, Feil IK, Lijnema TH, Hol WGJ, Agsteribbe E, Wilschut J. Mutants of the *Escherichia coli* Heat-Labile enterotoxin with reduced ADP-Ribosylation activity or no activity retain the immunogenic properties of the native holotoxin. *Infect Immun* 1996; 64: 5413-6.
37. Douce G, Fontana M, Pizza M, Rappuoli R, Dougan G. Intranasal immunogenicity and adjuvanticity of site-directed mutant derivatives of cholera toxin. *Infect Immun* 1997; 65: 2821-8.
38. Green EA, Botting C, Webb HM, Hirst TR, Randall RE. Construction, purification and immunogenicity of antigen-antibody-LTB complexes. *Vaccine* 1996; 14: 949-58.
39. Williams NA, Stasiuk LM, Nashar TO, Richards CM, Lang AK, Day MJ, Hirst TR. Prevention of autoimmune disease due to lymphocyte modulation by the B-subunit of *Escherichia coli* heat-labile enterotoxin. *Proc Natl Acad Sci USA* 1997; 94: 5290-5.
40. Czerkinsky C, Sun JB, Lebens M, Li BL, Rask C, Lindblad M, Holmgren J. Cholera toxin B-subunit as transmucosal carrier delivery and immunomodulating system for induction of antiinfectious and antipathological immunity. *Ann NY Acad Sci* 1996; 778: 185-93.
41. Sun JB, Holmgren J, Czerkinsky C. Cholera toxin B subunit – an efficient transmucosal carrier delivery system for induction of peripheral immunological tolerance. *Proc Natl Acad Sci USA* 1994; 91: 10795-9.
42. Sun JB, Rask C, Olsson T, Holmgren J, Czerkinsky C. Treatment of experimental autoimmune encephalomyelitis by feeding myelin basic protein conjugated to cholera-toxin-subunit. *Proc Natl Acad Sci USA* 1996; 93: 7196-201.
43. Bergerot I, Ploix C, Petersen J, Moulin V, Rask C, Fabien N, Lindbald M, Mayer A, Czerkinsky C, Holmgren J, Thivolet C. A cholera toxoid-insulin conjugate as an oral vaccine against spontaneous autoimmune diabetes. *Proc Natl Acad Sci USA* 1997; 94: 4610-4.
44. Rocken M, Racke M, Shevach EM. IL-4-induced immune deviation as antigen-specific threapy for inflammatory autoimmune disease. *Immunol Today* 1996; 17: 225-31.

Recent advances in the pathogenesis of gastrointestinal bacterial infections.
P. Rampal, P. Boquet, eds. John Libbey Eurotext, Paris © 1998, pp. 175-189.

Enterotoxins which induce apoptosis or protect against apoptosis in epithelial cells

Carla Fiorentini, Alessia Fabbri, Loredana Falzano

Department of Ultrastructures, Istituto Superiore di Sanità, Viale Regina Elena 299, 00161 Rome, Italy

In the past few years, increasing numbers of bacterial pathogens have been identified as mediators of apoptosis *in vitro* (for a review, see [1]). Activation of apoptosis might be an efficient way by which bacteria neutralize the first line of non-specific host defence mediated by professional phagocytes, such as macrophages and polymorphonuclear cells (PMNs). Strategies of activating cell death may be widespread, since not only bacteria themselves, but also exotoxins such as diphtheria toxin [2], *Bordetella pertussis* adenylate cyclase cyclolysin [3] and others, can induce apoptosis *in vitro*. Bacteria producing such toxins may obviously benefit from killing macrophages since doing so they prevent their own ingestion and therefore their destruction. By inducing apoptosis, pathogens can thus successfully initiate infection and thereby colonize the tissues. Another situation in which the killing of the host cells would be beneficial for bacteria may be the induction of apoptosis of epithelial cells. By means of such damaging events, a bacterial pathogen colonizing the gut can induce the epithelium to slough off, thus allowing clearance and microbial dissemination, as it has recently been suggested for *Pseudomonas aeruginosa* [4], which can induce apoptosis by exotoxin A [2].

In this chapter we deal with enterotoxins only, focalizing our attention on those toxins produced by enteric bacteria and which have been described to interfere with the apoptotic pathway in epithelial cells. Before detailing the effects of each single toxin, a short overview on apoptosis and its role in the intestine will be presented.

Apoptotic cell death

Apoptosis is a form of cell death that plays a major role during development, homeostasis, and in many diseases including cancer, acquired immunodeficency syndrome, and neurodegenerative disorders [5]. Apoptosis occurs through the activation of a cell-intrinsic suicide program. The basic machinery to carry out apoptosis appears to be present in essentially all mammalian cells at all times, but the activation of the suicide program is regulated by many different signals that originate from both inside and outside the cells. This type of regulation allows for the elimination of cells that have been produced in excess, developed improperly, or sustained genetic damage. As schematically shown in *figure 1*, apoptosis is a multi-phase process. After having received an external signal to undergo apoptosis, a cell enters a condemned phase in which it becomes committed to die. This stage varies in lenght and lacks notable morphological hallmarks. In the absence of external signals triggering a reprieve, the condamned cell ultimately engages the so-called execution phase, a cell-autonomous death pathway that takes care of its disassembly into apoptotic bodies [6]. During the execution phase, the caspase family of proteases is though to be activated and to cleave specific substrates rapidly leading to cell death [7]. The engulfment and degradation of dead cells by macrophages end the process.

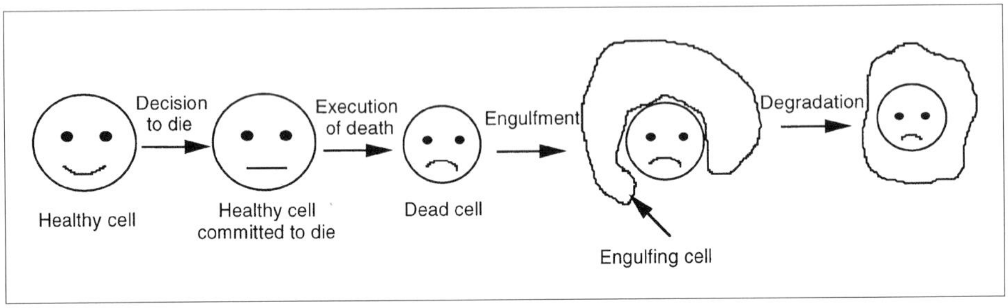

Figure 1. Schematic representation of the main steps of apoptosis.

Morphological alterations associated with apoptosis were largely detected by electron microscopy and include cell shrinkage, plasma and nuclear membrane blebbing, organelle relocalization and compaction, chromatin condensation and production of membrane-enclosed particles containing intracellular material known as "apoptotic bodies". By contrast, alterations typical of the alternative form of cell death, the necrosis, lead to rapid cellular disintegration, a process which typically involves cellular swelling, organelle dysfunction, mitochondrial collapse and the spillage of cellular contents into the extracellular environment. The lack of cellular debris generated by apoptotic cells appears to be important. Apoptotic cells display no obvious change in plasma membrane integrity, even while biochemical alterations are underway, allowing these cells to be cleared without triggering an inflammatory response. Furthermore, whereas individual cells undergo apoptotic cell death while surrounded by healthy neighbours, necrosis involves group of cells and has the deleterious end result of causing tissue inflammation [8].

Another cardinal feature of apoptosis is the cleavage of DNA into fragments, which are multiples of 180-200 basepairs, which corresponds to the size of a nucleosome. This produces a characteristic ladder appearance when DNA is subjected to agarose gel electrophoresis [9]. Often, this is preceded by DNA cleavage into large fragments 50 or 200 kilobases in size. By contrast, in necrosis the progressive disappearance of chromatin seen morphologically at a late stage of degeneration is accompanied by random DNA breakdown, as a diffuse smear appears in gels. In addition, apoptosis is often (but non exclusively) dependent upon ongoing protein and mRNA synthesis, as demonstrated by the observation that inhibitors (cycloheximide and actinomycin D) can prevent the death response in many instances [5].

The family of Bcl-2-related proteins plays key roles in the regulation of apoptosis and each family member can function to either block or promote cell death. Among the mammalian family members the most characterized are the antiapoptotic genes bcl-2 and bcl-X_L and proapoptotic gene bax. Bcl-2 localizes to the nuclear membrane, endoplasmic reticulum and the outer mitochondrial membrane; Bcl-X_L localizes to the outer membrane of mitochondria although present also in a soluble cytosolic form; Bax localization varies depending on its activity, this protein moving from the cytosol to the organelle membranes after induction of apoptosis [10]. The mechanism by which these molecules can affect the apoptotic process seems to be associated with heterodimerization among the family members. Bcl-2 proteins have also been described to control the alterations in mitochondrial permeability transition linked to membrane potential disruption which precede nuclear and plasma membrane changes [11].

Apoptosis of epithelial cells: the intestine as a model

Certain cell types need adhesion among cells as well as adhesion to an extracellular matrix in order to survive. For example, cells forming epithelia or endothelia easily undergo apoptosis once detached from the monolayer or when they loose contact with the neighbours. This type of apoptosis has been called by Frisch and Francis "anoikia" [12] which means "homeless". Lack of adhesion leads to anoikia and, on the other hand, the acquisition of anoikis resistance could facilitate anchorage-independent growth and, perhaps, transformation [13]. Thus, anoikia can be considered as a protective mechanism in those circumstances when the detachment of an "altered" cell triggers the self-killing, avoiding adhesion to an inappropriate tissue where it can resume growth. Although mechanisms by which adhesion to substrates controls cell proliferation and survival are not completely understood, integrin occupancy, cytoskeletal organization, cell spreading and the consequent change in cell shape are indicated as pivotal players [14].

The rational which led us to choose the intestine as a model for apoptosis in epithelial cells is that the toxins herein described are all produced by intestinal bacteria. Anoikia is of a great importance in the intestine because of the continuos renewal of cells and their need to be correctly located in the epithelium. In the small intestine, apoptosis can be observed in the crypts of healthy mice and humans, although the phenomenon interests an extremely small fraction of the total number of epithelial cells [15]. However, the cell death observed in the small intestine tends to be specifically located at the proposed site of stem cells, *i.e.* above the functional differentiated Paneth cells. This spontaneous apoptosis, which involves undamaged healthy cells, may act to eliminate those stem cells in excess of tissue requirements [15].

The levels of spontaneous apoptosis are significantly higher in the small intestine than in the large intestine. In a midcolon crypt, apoptotic cells are scattered througout the proliferative compartment without association with the proposed stem cell location. The antiapoptotic gene bcl-2 is usually expressed at the base of the crypts in the colons of mice and humans, suggesting a protective role against apoptosis efforted by bcl-2 expression in injured stem cells in the colon [15]. In the small intestine, the bcl-2 gene is, on the contrary, never expressed.

It is still controversial whether apoptosis is the mode of cell death leading to the removal of epithelial cells at the villus tip [16]. It is rare that cells in this region of the epithelium show the apoptotic morphological changes above described, although occasional apoptotic cells can be observed at the villus tip. Possibly, before the appearance of the classical apoptotic features, cells have first to loose adhesion contacts and be shed into the lumen [17]. Taking into account the above reported information, the intestinal epithelium provides unique advantages for studying apoptosis although more studies are required to fully understand the fate of intestinal cells.

However, most information on apoptosis (anoikia) in epithelial cells comes from observations obtained in cell cultures *in vitro*. Large numbers of studies have been focalized on the role of cell adhesion for the cell destiny. Cellular attachment of epithelial, endothelial and some tumor cells to the extracellular matrix through integrins promotes cell survival by inhibiting apoptosis [18]. Zhang *et al.* first showed [19] that integrin $\alpha5\beta1$ binding to fibronectin was particularly efficient at preventing cell death in serum-free medium. In this study, the $\alpha5$ integrin subunit cytoplasmic domain was shown to possibly regulate the expression of the cell death suppressor Bcl-2 [19]. Interactions of integrins with extracellular matrix proteins can activate integrin signal transducers such as the focal adhesion kinase (p^{125}FAK) which participates in the control of cell anchorage dependence. FAK can regulate anoikis in normal epithelial and endothelial cells and the conferral of anoikis resistance might be sufficient to transform certain epithelial cells [13].

Enterotoxins and apoptosis in epithelial cells

Bacteria which utilize apoptosis for expressing their virulence do so by undertaking different strategies, including either activation of apoptosis to destroy cells (professional phagocytes or epithelial cells) ot inhibition of host cell apoptosis, beneficial *in fine* for survival of intracellular pathogens [1]. Up to date no enterotoxins have been shown to interfere directly with proteins regulating the apoptotic pathway in epithelial cells. They all act on proteins belonging to the p21 Rho family inducing consequently a reorganization of the actin cytoskeleton *(figure 2)*.

Clostridium difficile toxin A

The anaerobic bacterium *Clostridium difficile* involved in the pathogenesis of antibiotic-associated diarrhoea and pseudomembranous colitis produces two large

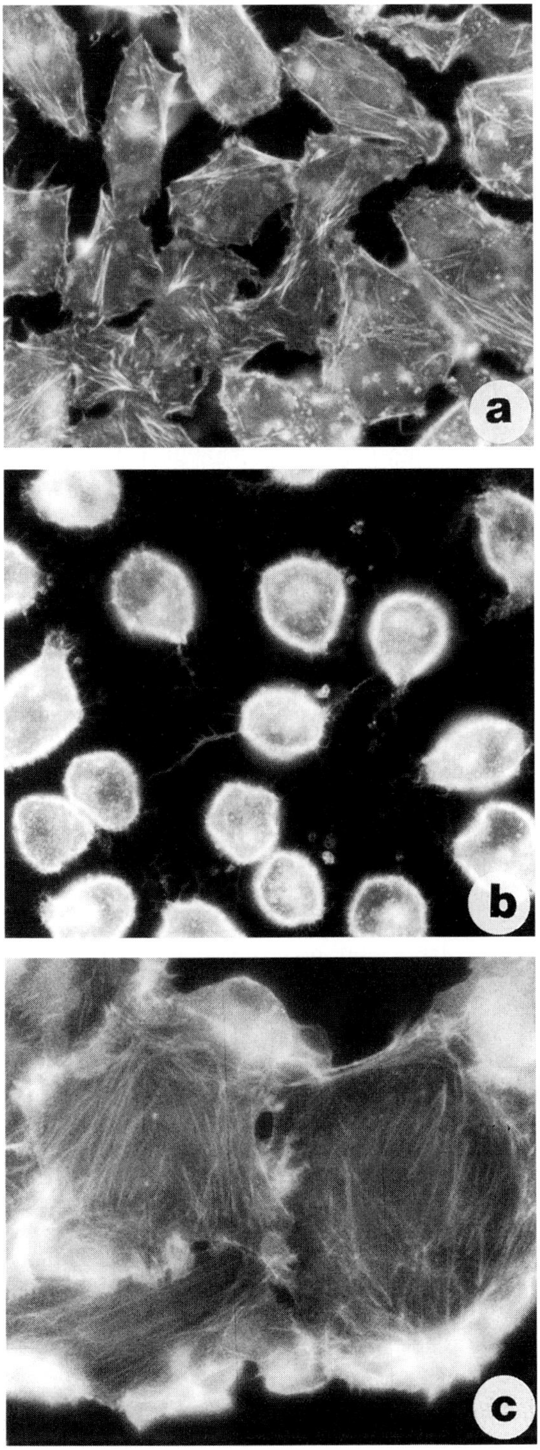

Figure 2. Actin cytoskeleton reorganization as induced by TCdB and CNF1 in epithelial cultured cells. Fluorescence micrographs of HEp-2 cells stained for F-actin detection. Control cells (a); cells treated with 3 ng/ml TCdB for 18 h (b) or 10^{-10} M CNF1 for 48 h (c). Note the breakdown of the actin network due to TCdB and the assembly of actin into prominent ruffles and stress fibers upon exposure to CNF1.

single-chain protein exotoxins: toxin A (TCdA), a cytotoxic enterotoxin and toxin B (TCdB), a more potent cytotoxin without enterotoxic activity [20]. After internalization into cells by endocytosis, their potent cytotoxicity results *in vitro* in the disaggregation of the actin cytoskeleton leading to the rounding up of the cell body. TCdA and TCdB are monoglucosyltransferases which catalyse the incorporation of glucose moiety into Thr 37 of RhoA or Thr 35 of both Rac and Cdc42 [21, 22], small GTP-binding proteins of the Rho family, involved in the regulation of actin assembly [23]. This modification renders Rho, Rac and Cdc42 inactive thereby losing their properties to induce actin polymerization and filaments bundling. Inactivation of Rho, Rac and Cdc42 by glucosylation appears to be the molecular mechanism by which *C. difficile* toxins mediate cytotoxic effects in cells.

The first study, dealing with TCdA and apoptosis was conducted by us on intestinal cultured crypt cells, IEC-6 cells *(figure 3)*. Although we did not refer to apoptosis, cells exposed to the toxin clearly exhibited the typical morphological features of such type of cell death [24]. As viewed by scanning electron microscopy, all TCdA-treated cells retracted the cell body and underwent rounding up. Moreover, in a sizable percentage of cells surface blebbing was clearly evident. Interestingly, the blebbing phenomenon was strictly correlated to apoptosis, blebbing cells displaying nuclear fragmentation by Hoechst staining. Thin-section transmission electron micrographs of TCdA-treated IEC-6 cells clearly showed two subpopulations, one devoid of surface blebs, characterized by nuclear polarization and by a slight dilatation of the rough endoplasmic reticulum; the other one, with surface blebs, showed dramatic morphological changes such as chromatin marginalization and condensation with a pycnotic appearance of the nuclei and a remarkable dilatation and vesiculation of the rough endoplasmic reticulum. In these cells, the bleb matrix contained ribosomes, normal and vesicular rough endoplasmic reticulum and mitochondria. It has to be underlined that all the above reported changes were observed in cells still adhering to the substrate. Thus, in this case, cell blebbing is a clear marker of apoptosis. Apoptotic membrane blebbing has been very recently reported as inhibited by inactivation of Rho and due to acto-myosin contraction [25], a process known to involve this small G protein [26]. In this last report, however, inactivation of Rho was followed by membrane blebbing. Further studies are now in progress to solve this controversial.

Apoptosis in intestinal cells induced by TCdA has been reported more recently by Mahida and coworkers [27]. In this study, however, apoptosis was detected only in cells which had already lost their interactions with the substrate, thus undergoing anoikia. The authors dealt with enterocytes and crypt cell lines and showed that both underwent cell retraction and rounding after TCdA exposure (although at different times, the first type of cells being more sensitive than the second type, *i.e.* the effects appeared at least 24 h before in enterocytes than in crypt cells). Cells in detached monolayers initially remained viable while adherent to each other as viewed by trypan blue exclusion [27]. The number of floating individual cells increased with time of exposure to TCdA and such cells were not capable of excluding the dye. Transmission electron microscopy studies were in keeping with the above reported findings, since cells in the detached monolayers ultrastructurally appeared viable while adhering to each other. Prolonging the time of exposure to the toxin,

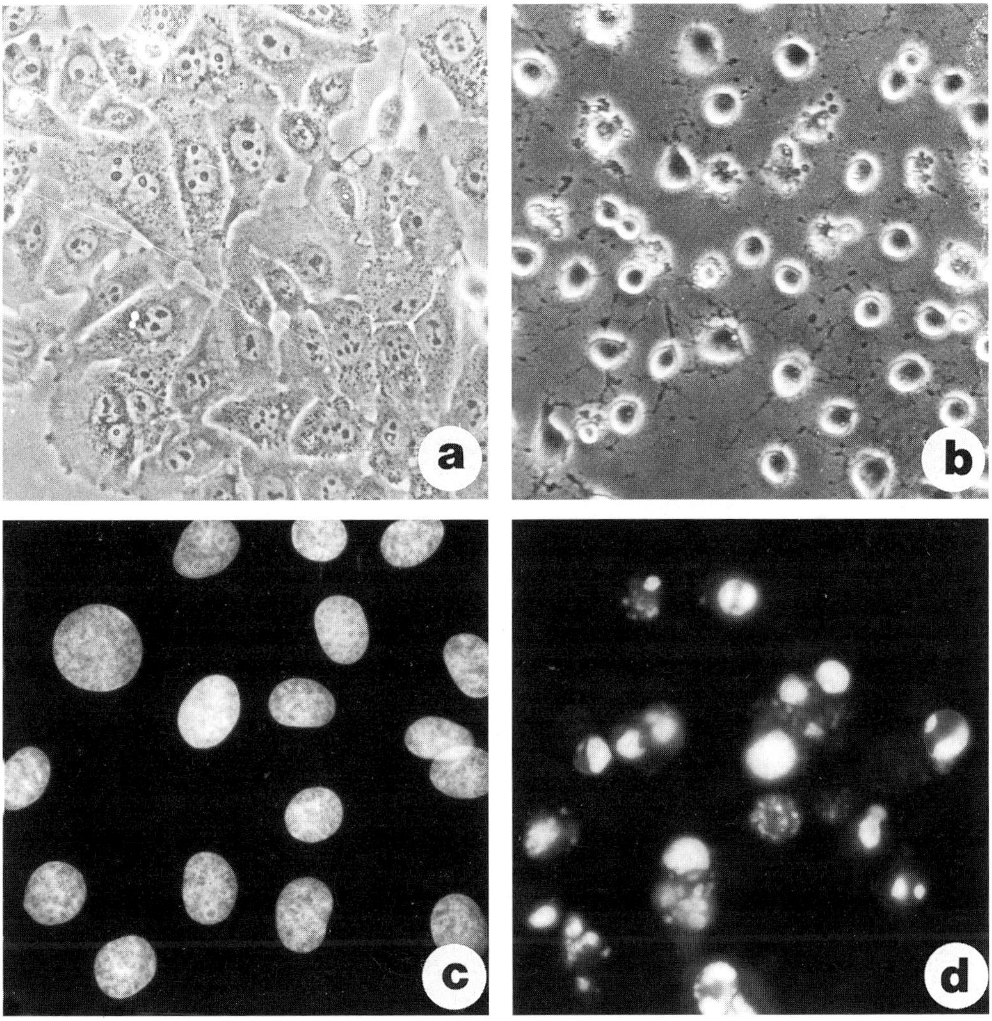

Figure 3. TCdB induces apoptosis in intestinal epithelial cells. Phase contrast micrographs (a, b) and nuclear staining by the fluorescent probe Hoechst (c, d) of IEC-6 cells. Control cells (a, c) and cells exposed to 3 ng/ml TCdB for 18 h (b, d). Note the rounding up of the cell body, the membrane blebbing, the chromatin condensation and fragmentation typical of apoptosis in cells treated with the toxin.

an increasing number of smaller individual cells in suspension appeared and interestingly they showed apoptotic features. In these cells, while the cell membrane and many cytoplasmic organelles retained integrity, the nuclei were characteristically broken into discrete spherical structures containing dense chromatin. Subsequently, the cells broke into discrete membrane-bound apoptotic bodies with eventual complete disintegration into cellular debris. An identical sequence of events was found when a human colonic mucosa in organ colture was used, suggesting that this should be the action of the toxin *in vivo* [27]. In such a model, identical results were obtained when cells where detached with EDTA, leaving open the question whether the apoptotic effect was due to the direct action of the toxin or ony the consequence of the cell anchorage loss.

Interestingly, in the same report [27], detached colonic epithelial cells were shown to be able to produce IL-8 during the first 24 h of exposure to TCdA. Apoptosis may thus allow injured epithelial cells to respond by secreting molecules which in turn will interact with other cells to initiate a systemic protective response.

Clostridium difficile toxin B

The first observation on TCdB as inducer of cell death was reported in 1990 [28]. The toxin, able to induce rounding up and blebbing in different cell lines, also caused morphological effects on epithelial cells strongly resembling apoptotic changes. The blebbing phenomenon was investigated by several tecniques, particularly referring to its significance as a sign of stress and in relationships with the cell cytoskeleton [28]. Even though the world "apoptosis" did not appear in that report, some of the micrographs (as viewed today) clearly showed characteristic apoptotic features *(figure 4)*. We have thus undertaken a new study on this topic, using the same intestinal cell system (IEC-6) which undergoes apoptosis upon exposure to TCdA [24]. TCdB showed the same capability of provoking apoptotic cell death, clear morphological changes such as chromatin condensation and fragmentation being evident in a significant percentage of cells [29]. Moreover, typical flow cytometric hallmarks of apoptosis were detected, a sub-G1 hypodiploid peak, due to the reduced amount of DNA per cell being evident after 18 and 48 h of TCdB treatment. According to the morphological observations, flow cytometric studies showed that the apoptotic response was linked to toxin exposure time, reaching about 33% of cells after 48 h treatment [29].

Apoptosis is a toxin dose- and time-dependent process, not simply due to the actin-disrupting effect of TCdB nor to the subsequent impairment of cell anchorage. Rather, the inhibition of proteins belonging to the Rho family due to TCdB seems to play a role in the induction of apoptosis in intestinal cells. The origin of cells and the growth rate may also represent relevant cofactors in such a response. Moreover, cells seemed to counteract the apoptotic response induced by TCdB with newly synthesized proteins, since the inhibition of protein synthesis allowed the appearence of a more potent apoptotic response [29]. Preliminary results from our group showed that the intracellular content of proteins belonging to the Bcl-2 family was not modified by toxin treatment. Studies are now in progress in our laboratory to address these questions.

Clostridium botulinum exoenzyme C3

Although C3 is not a real enterotoxin and its role as apoptotic inducer has not been explored on epithelial cells, we have included it in this chapter because C3 is actually the main reagent to explore the various intracellular functions of Rho. In this respect, it is becoming evident that this regulatory G protein is involved in the control of apoptosis.

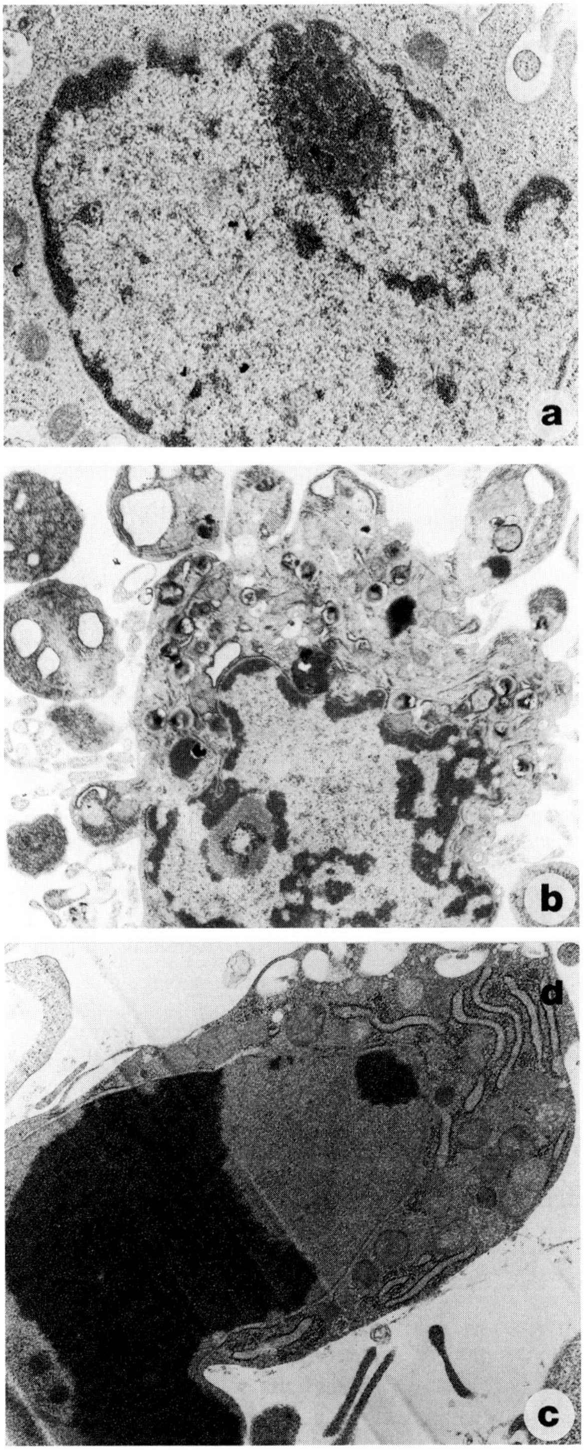

Figure 4. Ultrastructural features of apoptotic IEC-6 cells upon exposure to TCdA. Transmission electron micrographs of (a) control cells and (b, c) treated-cells. Cells showing the typical features of apoptosis were characterized by membrane blebbing, marginalization and/or condensation of chromatin and remarkable dilatation and vesiculation of the endoplasmic reticulum.

C. botulinum C3 is known to ADP-ribosylate the small GTP-binding protein Rho at Asn41, a modification that functionally inactivates Rho [30]. C3 has been shown to induce apoptosis in particular situations and in particular systems, mostly as inhibitor of the Rho GTP-binding protein. Using a Sindbis virus-based transient gene expression system, Moorman *et al.* [31] studied the role of Rho in murine EL4 T lymphoma cells. By such system, C3 expressed intracellularly in intact lymphocytes, led to a rapid and efficient inactivation of virtually all endogenous Rho. Using propidium iodide staining, they observed that, infected cells underwent inhibition of cytokinesis, the majority of them containing two or more nuclei. Quantification of DNA content by flow cytometry allowed the identification of a cell population with an amount of DNA 8N and 16N. Thus cell cycle progression continued despite the inhibition of cytokinesis. Moreover, following dsSIN:C3 infection, Moorman and colleagues showed evidence of apoptosis, including nuclear condensation, formation of apoptotic bodies and DNA fragmentation evidenced by a ladder on agarose gel electrophoresis. The activation of apoptosis was independent of multinucleate cell formation. In fact, when 5-Fura was used to inhibit cell cycle progression and thus multinucleation, dsSIN:C3 infection still caused marked apoptosis. Such an apoptotic response seemed to be caused by the C3-mediated inactivation of Rho protein.

Very recently Henning *et al.* [32] have inactivated Rho function in the thymus by targeting a transgene encoding C3 transferase. While no discernible effects was evident on positive and negative selection process in the thymus (all populations with different surface markers being found at the different stages) a decrease in cell number was clearly observed. In fact, the number of thymocytes traversing the cell cycle in rho- thymi was reduced and the levels of apoptotic cells was found to be increased. This suggested that thymocyte differentiation was able to procede also in the absence of functional Rho. The Rho activity seemed, however, to be essential for thymocyte subsets maintenance and proliferative expansion.

Escherichia coli cytotoxic necrotizing factor 1

The cytotoxic necrotizing factor 1 (CNF1) is a 110 kDa protein toxin produced by certain enterotoxigenic and uropathogenic *E. coli* strains. After internalization into cells by endocytosis [33], CNF1 exerts its activity by bundling actin filaments and mainly inducing stress fibers accumulation [34]. It has recently been demonstrated that CNF1 enzymatic activity consists in the deamidation of the p21 Rho glutamin 63 which results in a mutation into glutamic acid [35, 36]. The p21 Rho GTP-binding protein is known to be involved in the actin assembly regulation and the modification induced by CNF1 on Rho leads to the permanent activation of the G protein. This therefore leads to the subsequent activation of a number of kinases in cells, particularly the ser/thr kinase Rho-kinase (Rock) [37, 38] and seems to be at the basis of the prominent reorganization of the actin cytoskeleton due to CNF1. Such changes induced by CNF1 may influence and modify some functional cellular properties. We have indeed reported that this toxin provokes an aspecific phagocytic-like behaviour in epithelial cells, allowing non-invasive bacteria to be taken up and to multiply intracellularly [33].

Strictly correlated with this finding is the fact that CNF1 can protect cells against apoptosis induced by certain stimuli such as ultraviolet radiation (UVB) [39]. As shown in *figure 5*, while cells exposed to UVB displayed cell retraction, rounding, alteration of surface structures and nuclei with fragmented and condensed chromatin, all markers of apoptosis, cells challenged with CNF1 for at least 48 h before UVB irradiation were significantly protected from all these effects. In addition, CNF1 was capable of significantly protecting cells by the actin disrupting effects due to UVB. Between cellular events downstream the activation of Rho by CNF1 and involved in protection against apoptosis, we found that Bcl-2 family proteins level and mitochondrial homeostasis played an important role. We have indeed shown that CNF1 was capable of reducing the mitochondrial membrane depolarization induced by UVB and to modulate the intracellular expression of some bcl-2 related proteins. In particular, the amount of death antagonist Bcl-2 and Bcl-X_L increased following exposure to CNF1 while the amount of the death agonist Bax remained substantially unchanged [40]. Mitochondria and the bcl-2 family proteins have an essential role in apoptosis [11, 41, 42] and they are linked one to each other. Thus, our results suggested that CNF1, by modulating the expression of proteins of Bcl-2 family (probably *via* Rho activation), may operate on one of the main regulatory systems which drive a cell towards death or survival: the mitochondrial function.

When the correlation between the induction of phagocytic activity and the protection of apoptosis was studied, we found that while the ability of ingesting bacteria increased by time of CNF1 exposure, the percentage of apoptotic cells decreased. The plateau for both activities was reached after 48 h. Thus, our results showed a significant inverse correlation between the two phenomena, suggesting that they could be part of a pathogenic mechanism used by bacteria [39]. In fact, once inside a cell, microorganisms need this cell to be alive and functionally active for their own multiplication. It would be deleterious, therefore, if the epithelial cell turns on apoptosis during the bacterial invasion.

Conclusions

Apoptosis is clearly important in the pathogenicity of various infectious diseases and certain bacterial pathogens have evolved ways to induce eukaryotic cell death using protein toxins as potent weapons. Some enterotoxins, as above reported, may interfere with the apoptotic pathway in epithelial cells. Effects induced by *C. difficile* toxins in intestinal cells appear to be relevant since the gut is the actual target of TCdA and TCdB in experimental animals. Although the role played by apoptosis in the pathogenicity of both toxins *in vivo* is not clear, we can speculate that intestinal cells undergoing apoptosis upon exposure to them can then liberate cytokines capable of mediating an inflammatory process. Such inflammation could be reinforced by the actin-disrupting effect of the toxins on macrophages which are consequently impaired in their migration and unable to phagocytose apoptotic cells before they lyse.

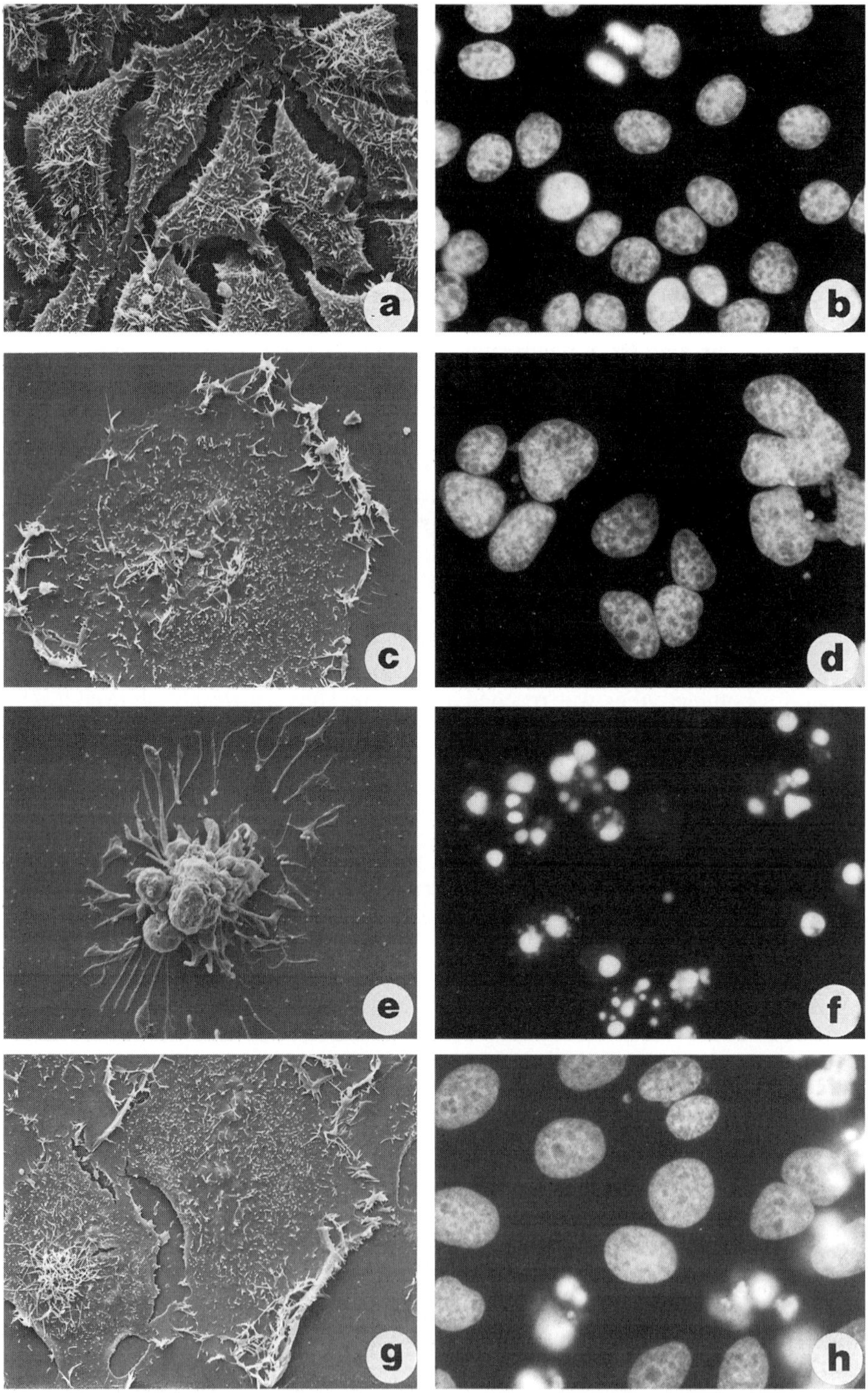
a
b
c
d
e
f
g
h

On the other hand, inhibition of host cell apoptosis may represent a beneficial strategy for surviving inside mammalian cells. CNF1 hinders the apoptotic cell death in epithelial cells and, furthermore, induces an aspecific phagocytic-like activity in non-professional phagocytes, *i.e.* epithelial cells. Taken together these events may represent a mechanism used by pathogenic CNF1-producing *E. coli* to enter cells, multiply and be transcytosed through the epithelium to the blood stream. During the bacterial invasion, the epithelial cell must be alive and functionally active without turning on apoptosis. Moreover, more than a way to enter cells, CNF1 could fournish to the bacterium a protected "niche" from external insults. All these processes may favour a successful infectious process. In our view, however, inhibition of the "clean" death process, *i.e.* apoptosis, may consequently rise the possibility that cells *forced* to survive by CNF1 activity undergo changes in their proliferative program, thus raising the possibility of cellular transformation.

In the intestine, the importance of apoptosis mainly lies in its role in carcinogenesis and hence the promise of treatment for cancer. It is now believed that colorectal cancer comes from a series of mutations of specific oncogenes and tumor suppressor genes. Some of these genes act by regulating apoptosis. For example, the different expression of the anti-apoptotic gene *bcl-2* in the intestinal cells (positive at the base of colonic crypts and absent in the small intestine) can partially explain the difference in the tendency of small and large intestinal epithelium to undergo apoptosis. The full understanding of factors that regulate apoptosis may allow the cell fate manipulation with the final goal of developing therapies for the treatment of cancer.

◄ **Figure 5.** CNF1 prevents UVB-induced apoptosis in epithelial cells. Micrographs of HEp-2 cells as viewed by scanning electron microscopy (on the left) and fluorescence microscopy upon Hoechst 33.258 staining (on the right). Control cells (a, b); cells treated with 10^{-10} M CNF1 for 48 h (c, d); UVB-treated cells (e, f); cells treated first with CNF1 and then with UVB (g, h). Note that CNF1 counteracts both the radiation-induced rounding up and the chromatin clumping.

References

1. Zychinsky A, Sansonetti P. Apoptosis in bacterial pathogenesis. *J Clin Invest* 1997; 100: 493-6.
2. Kochi SK, Collier RJ. DNA fragmentation and cytolysis in U937 cells treated with diphtheria toxin or other inhibitors of protein synthesis. *Exp Cell Sci* 1993; 208: 296-302.
3. Khelef N, Zychlinsky A, Guiso N. *Bordetella pertussis* induces apoptosis in macrophages: role of adenylate cyclase-hemolysin. *Infect Immun* 1993; 61: 4064-71.
4. Pier G, Grout M, Zaidi T, Olsen J, Johnson L, Yankaskas J, Goldberg J. Role of mutant CFTR in hypersusceptibility of cystic fibrosis patients to lung infections. *Science (Wash. DC)* 1996; 271: 64-7.
5. Orrenius S. Apoptosis: molecular mechanisms and implications for human disease. *J Int Med* 1995; 237: 529-36.
6. Martins LM, Earnshaw WC. Apoptosis: alive and kicking in 1997. *Trends Cell Biol* 1997; 7: 111-4.
7. Nicholson, Thornberry. Caspases: killer proteases. *Trends Biochem Sci* 1997, 22: 299-306.
8. McConkey, DJ, Zhivotovsky B, Orrenius S. *Molecular aspects of medicine: apoptosis- molecular mechanisms and biomedical implications.* Oxford: Elsevier Science Ltd, 1996: 17: 1-170.
9. Wyllie AH. Glucocorticoid-induced thymocyte apoptosis is associated with endogenous endonuclease activation. *Nature* 1980; 284: 555.
10. Wolter KG, Hsu YT, Smith CL, Nechushtan A, Xi XG, Youle RJ. Movement of Bax from the cytosol to mitochondria during apoptosis. *J Cell Biol* 1997; 139: 1281-92.
11. Kroemer G. The proto-oncogene Bcl-2 and its role in regulating apoptosis. *Nature Med* 1997; 3: 614-20.
12. Frish SM, Francis H. Disruption of epithelial cell-matrix interactions induce apoptosis. *J Cell Biol* 1994; 124: 619-26.
13. Frish SM, Vuori K, Rouslahti E, Chan-Hui PY. Control of adhesion-dependent cell survival by focal adhesion kinase. *J Cell Biol* 1996, 134: 793-9.
14. Rouslahti E. Stretching is good for a cell. *Science* 1997; 276: 1345-6.
15. Potten CS. Epithelial cell growth and differentiation II. Intestinal apoptosis. *Am J Physiol* 1997; 273: G253-257.
16. Iwanaga T, Han H, Adachi K, Fujita T. A novel mechanism for disposing of effete epithelial cells in the small intestine of guinea pigs. *Gastroenterology* 1993; 105: 1089- 97.
17. Watson AJM. Necrosis and apoptosis in the gastrointestinal tract. *Gut* 1995; 37: 165-7.
18. Meredith JE Jr, Schwartz MA. Integrins, adhesion and apoptosis. *Trends Cell Biol* 1997; 7: 146-50.
19. Zhang Z, Vuori K, Reed JC, Rouslahti E. The $\alpha 5\beta 1$ integrin supports survival of cells on fibronectin and up-regulates Bcl-2 expression. *Proc Natl Acad Sci USA* 1995; 6161-5.
20. Thelestam M, Florin I, Olarte EC. *Clostridium difficile* toxins. In: Aktories K, ed. *Bacterial toxin.* Weinheim: Chapman & Hall, 1997: 141-58.
21. Just I, Selzer J, Wilm M, von Eichel-Streiber C, Mann M, Aktories K. Glycosylation of rho proteins by *Clostridium difficile* toxin B. *Nature* 1995; 375: 500-3.
22. Just I, Selzer M, Rex J, von Eichel-Streiber C, Mann M, Aktories K. The enterotoxin from *Clostridium difficile* (ToxA) monoglucosylates the Rho protein. *J Biol Chem* 1995; 270: 13392-6.
23. Hall A. Rho GTPases and the actin cytoskeleton. *Science* 1998; 279: 509-14.
24. Fiorentini C, Donelli G, Nicotera P, Thelestam M. *Clostridium difficile* toxin A elicits Ca^{+2}-independent cytotoxic effects in cultured normal rat crypt cells. *Infect Immun* 1993; 61: 3988-93.

25. Mills JC, Stone NL, Erhardt J, Pittman RN. Apoptotic membrane blebbing is regulated by myosin light chain phosphorylation. *J Cell Biol* 1998; 40: 627-36.
26. Kimura K, Ito M, Amano M, Chihara K, Fukuta Y, Nakafuku M, Yamamori B, Feng J, Nakano T, Okawa K, Iwamatsu A, Kaibuchi K. Regulation of myosin phosphatase by Rho and Rho associated kinase (Rho-kinase). *Science* 1996; 273: 245-8.
27. Mahida YR, Makh S, Hyde S, Gray T, Borriello SP. Effect of *Clostridium difficile* toxin A on human intestinal epithelial cells: induction of interleukin 8 production and apoptosis after cell detachment. *Gut* 1996; 38: 337-47.
28. Malorni W, Fiorentini C, Paradisi S, Giuliano M, Mastrantonio P, Donelli G. Surface blebbing and cytoskeletal changes induced *in vitro* by toxin B from *Clostridium difficile*: an immunochemical and ultrastructural study. *Exp Mol Pathol* 1990; 52: 340-56.
29. Fiorentini C, Fabbri A, Falzano L, Fattorossi A, Matarrese P, Rivabene R, Donelli G. *Clostridium difficile* toxin B induces apoptosis in intestinal cultured cells. *Infect Immun* 1998 (in press).
30. Chardin P, Boquet P, Madaule P, Popoff MR, Rubin EJ, Gill DM. The mammalian G protein rho C is ADP-ribisylated by Clostridium botulinum exoenzyme C3 and affects actin microfilament in Vero cells. *EMBO J* 1989; 8: 1087.
31. Moorman, JP, DA Bobak, Hahn CS. Inactivation of the small GTP binding protein Rho induces multinucleate cell formation and apoptosis in murine T lymphoma EL4. *J Immunol* 1996; 156: 4146-53.
32. Henning SW, Galandrini R, Hall A, Cantrell DA. The GTPase Rho has a critical regulatory role in thymus development. *EMBO J* 1997; 16: 2397-407.
33. Falzano L, Fiorentini C, Donelli G, Michel E, Kocks C, Cossart P, Cabanié L, Oswald E, Boquet P. Induction of phagocytic behaviour in human epithelial cells by *Escherichia coli* Cytotoxic Necrotizing Factor type 1. *Mol Microbiol* 1993; 9: 1247-54.
34. Fiorentini C, Arancia G, Caprioli A, FalboV, Ruggeri FM, Donelli G. Cytoskeletal changes induced in Hep-2 cells by cytotoxic necrotizing factor of *Escherichia coli. Toxicon* 1988; 26: 1047-56.
35. Flatau G, Lemichez E, Gauthier M, Chardin P, Paris S, Fiorentini C, Boquet P. Toxin-induced activation of the G protein p21 Rho by deamidation of glutamine. *Nature* 1997; 387: 729-33.
36. Schmidt G, Sehr P, Wilm M, Selzer J, Mann M, Aktories K. Glu 63 of Rho is deaminated by *Escherichia coli* cytotoxic necrotizing factor -1. *Nature* 1997; 387: 725-9.
37. Fiorentini C, Fabbri A, Flatau G, Donelli G, Matarrese P, Lemichez E, Falzano L, Boquet P. *Escherichia coli* cytotoxic necrotizing factor 1 (CNF1): a toxin which activates the Rho GTPase. *J Biol Chem* 1997; 272: 19532-7.
38. Lacerda HM, Pullinger GD, Lax AJ, Rozengurt E. Cytotoxic necrotizing factor 1 from *Escherichia coli* and dermonecrotic toxin from *Bordetella bronchiseptica* induce p21 (rho)-dependent tyrosine phosphorilation of focal adhesion kinase and paxillin in Swiss 3T3 cells. *J Biol Chem* 1997; 272: 9587-96.
39. Fiorentini C, Fabbri A, Matarrese P, Falzano L, Boquet P, Malorni W. Hinderance of apoptosis and phagocytic behaviour induced by *E. coli* necrotizing factor 1 (CNF1): two related activities in epithelial cells. *Biochem Biophys Res Comm* 1997; 241: 341-6.
40. Fiorentini C, Matarrese P, Straface E, Falzano L, Fabbri A, Donelli G, Cossarizza A, Boquet P, Malorni W. Toxin-induced activation of Rho GTP-binding protein increases Bcl-2 expression and influences mitochondrial homeostasis. *Exp Cell Res* 1998 ; in press.
41. Kluck RM, Bossy-Wetzel E, Green DR, Newmeyer DD. The release of cytochrome c from mitochondria: a primary site for Bcl-2 regulation of apoptosis. *Science* 1997 275: 1132-6.
42. Reed JC. Double identity for proteins of the bcl-2 family. *Nature* 1997; 387: 773-6.

Recent advances in the pathogenesis of gastrointestinal bacterial infections.
P. Rampal, P. Boquet, eds. John Libbey Eurotext, Paris © 1998, pp. 191-203.

Enterotoxins and the enteric nervous system

Michael J.G. Farthing

Digestive Diseases Research Centre, St Bartholomew's & The Royal London School of Medicine & Dentistry, Turner Street, London, UK

Enterotoxin producing bacteria still constitute an important cause of diarrhoeal disease morbidity and mortality worldwide. Although cholera and enterotoxigenic *E. coli* are primarily infections of the developing world, exterotoxin producing bacteria are also found in industrialised countries including *Clostridium difficile, Campylobacter* spp. And enteroaggregative *E. coli.* Enterotoxin producing organisms are responsible for acute watery diarrhoea of varying severity ranging from cholera, in which intestinal losses may reach 1 litre/h, to milder forms of enterotoxigenic *E. coli* diarrhoea such as occurs commonly in travellers.
Enterotoxins are one of a number of virulence factors possessed by enteropathogenic bacteria which cause diarrhoeal disease [1]. Secretory enterotoxins such as cholera toxin and *E. coli* heat labile (LT) and heat stable (ST) toxins produce diarrhoea without inducing morphologic damage in the small or large intestine. Although it has been thought for many years that these toxins act directly on the enterocyte to activate intracellular secretory pathways and in some instances simultaneously inhibit sodium and chloride ion absorption, it is now evident that other pathogenetic pathways are involved including the release of endogenous secretagogues and the activation of secretory reflexes within the enteric nervous system. Indeed there is increasing evidence that the enteric nervous system is involved both in the physiologic control of basal and food stimulated absorption and secretion and also in a variety of pathologic situations notably acute infective diarrhoea.

Role of the enteric nervous system in intestinal secretion and absorption

Anatomy of the enteric nervous system

The enteric nervous system functions independently of the central nervous system but is connected to it through parasympathetic and sympathetic afferent and efferent neurones which assemble in the central nervous system as the central autonomic neural network [2, 3]. Cell bodies of enteric neurones are grouped together as ganglia connected by bundles of nerve processes which constitute two major plexuses, the myenteric plexus located between the circular and longitudinal muscles of the gut and the submucosal plexus located in submucosa between the circular muscle layer and the muscularis mucosae. The myenteric plexus is predominantly involved in the motor control of the gut but in addition provides secretomotor innervation to the mucosa. The submucosal plexus innervates the gut epithelium and has a central role in the control of secretory processes. In addition to the enteric neural network, other cell types are involved in the mediation of the actions of the enteric nervous system. Enteric glial cells, which are the intestinal counterpart of astrocytes in the central nervous system, are able to produce cytokines and express MHC class II antigens on exposure to cytokines, suggesting a role in modulating inflammatory processes. Enteric neurones may also influence effector systems indirectly by interaction with cells of the immune system, particularly mast cells. A population of non-neural cells, the interstitial cells of Cajal, serve as pacemakers for gut motor activity but have recently been shown to influence secretory processes in the gut through neuronal influences on mast cells.

Neurones within the enteric nervous system are classified as intrinsic afferent neurones, interneurones and motor or secretory neurones *(figure 1)*. The enteric nervous system functions through a variety of neurotransmitters of which more than twenty have been proposed *(table I)*. Confirmation of neurotransmitter function has however, only been confirmed for a relatively limited number of these substances, notably acetylcholine, γ aminobutyric acid (GABA), substance P, vasoactive intestinal polypeptide (VIP) and nitric oxide (NO). It is likely that neurotransmitter function will be confirmed for other putative neurotransmitters notably calcitonin gene-related peptide (CGRP) and neuropeptide Y. Although eight morpholocial forms of neurone have been identified in the enteric nervous system, two forms predominate, namely type I which have a single, long axon and numerous short club-shaped dendrites and type II neurones which are multi-polar possessing many long, smooth processes.

Submucosal plexus neurones are predominantly cholinergic or vasoactive intestinal peptidergic. However, cholinergic neurones may be further subdivided on the basis of their content of secondary peptides such as substance P, somatostatin, cholecystokinin and neuropeptide Y. Neurones in the myenteric ganglia are predominantly peptidergic, containing substance P, encephalins and 5-hydroxytyptamine (5-HT). These neurones project from the myenteric plexus, interacting with the submucosal plexus and the basolateral membrane of epithelial cells. Neural receptors for substance P, encephalins and 5-HT, as well as acetylcholine, catecholamines, ATP and vasoactive intestinal peptide are found in submucosal ganglia.

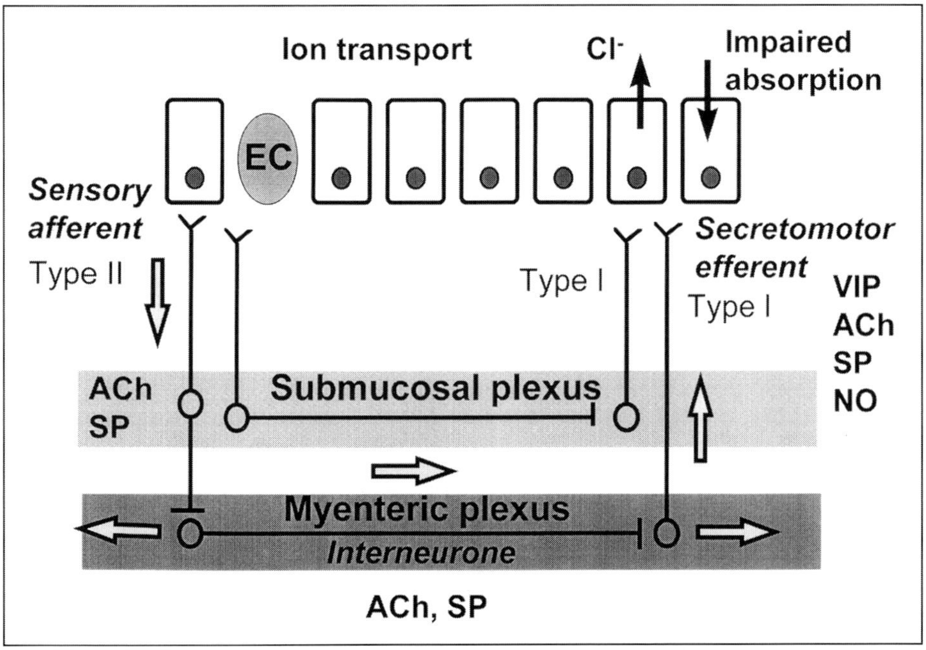

Figure 1. Role of the enteric nervous system in intestinal ion transport. The neural reflex consists of a type II neurone sensory afferent (probably cholinergic and/or substance pergic), an interneurone (probably cholinergic and/or substance pergic) and a type I secretomotor efferent (variety of proposed neurotransmitters). In addition to this local neural reflex, there may be cephalic and aboral neural transmission originating from this local reflex.
EC, enterochromaffin cell; ACh, acetylcholine; SP, substance P; VIP, vasoactive intestinal peptide; NO, nitric oxide.

Transport physiology

Activation of enteric nerves by electrical field stimulation was the first experimental intervention that clearly showed a role for the enteric nervous system in intestinal ion transport processes [4]. The increase in short-circuit current induced by electrical field stimulation was partially blocked by atropine and completely abolished by the neurotoxin, tetrodotoxin. Further studies clearly showed that the secretory state related to luminal distension and feeding were mediated at least in part by the enteric nervous system, with the involvement of neurotransmitters such as substance P and acetylcholine, and also the release of 5-HT from enterochromaffin cells [5-7]. More recently it has been shown that capsaicin sensitive primary afferents modulate nutrient absorption which has been confirmed experimentally *in vitro* with the amino acid, alanine [8]. It is thought that this effect is mediated through neuropeptide neurotransmitters such as VIP, substance P and CGRP.

The role of NO as a neurotransmitter in modulating absorptive and secretory processes remains controversial [9]. Nitrergic nerves have been identified in the submucosa in mammalian intestine, indicating that they may have a role in regulating electrolyte and water transport across the intestinal epithelium. However, *in vitro* and *in vivo* studies have produced conflicting results suggesting that under basal conditions, NO is pro-absorptive although in pathophysiological situations when present in excess, it may be pro-secretory [10-12]. Other neurotransmitters such as GABA and pituitary adenylate cyclase activating polypeptide (PACAP), a putative neurotransmitter in the enteric nervous system with close sequence homology with both VIP and its related pro-secretory peptide PHI, have also been implicated in the control of absorptive and secretory processes in the gut.

Table I. Established and putative neurotransmitters in the enteric nervous system

Amines	**Peptides**
* Acetylcholine	+ Calcitonin gene-related peptide (CGRP)
* Noradrenaline	Cholecystokinin (CCK)
5-hydroxytryptamine (5-HT)	Gastrin-releasing peptide (GRP)
	* Neuropeptide Y (NPY)
Amino acids	Neurotensin
* γ-aminobutyric acid (GABA)	Opioids
	Peptide YY (PYY)
	Pituitary adenylyl cyclase-activating peptide (PACAP)
Purines	* Somatostatin
ATP	* Substance P
	* Vasoactive intestinal polypeptide (VIP)
Gases	
* Nitric oxide	
Carbon monoxide	

* Neurotransmitter status established
+ Probable neurotransmitter

Bacterial enterotoxins

Bacterial enteropathogens rely on a number of virulence factors to colonise the mammalian intestine and produce diarrhoeal disease. These include (i) **adhesins** which are lectin-like molecules which mediate adherence to the enterocyte microvillous membrane, (ii) **invasins** which are bacterial proteins which mediate the invasion process usually by subverting cytoskeletal function of the host epithelial cell, (iii) **cytotoxins** which may be delivered intra or extracellularly producing epithelial cell death and (iv) **enterotoxins** which are usually secreted into the intestinal lumen and can both induce active ion secretion and inhibit ion absorption by the enterocyte *(table II)*. Enterotoxigenic diarrhoea is characterised by its watery nature, its relatively high sodium and chloride content and a lack of any macro or microscopic damage to the intestinal epithelium.

Classic modes of action

The most widely studied enterotoxin, cholera toxin and the closely related *E. coli* LT are ADP-ribosylating toxins which activate the enzyme adenylate cyclase with a resulting increase in intracellular cyclic AMP [1]. cAMP then activates a secretory cascade involving protein kinase A, protein phosphorylation and the opening of chloride channels in the apical membrane of the enterocyte, predominantly those located in the crypts. cAMP also inhibits the action of the sodium/hydrogen exchanger and its associated anion exchanger in villous enterocytes, thereby inhibiting neutral sodium and chloride absorption. In addition, both calcium and calmodulin have been implicated in cholera toxin induced secretion as has the increased synthesis of pro-secretory prostaglandins such PGE_2 and $PGEF_{2\alpha}$ probably directly by enterocytes.

E. coli ST and the family of relatex toxins *(table II)* are structurally very different to the CT/LT family of enterotoxins being much smaller, heat stable and acting through an apical receptor which is directly linked to membrane bound guanylate cyclase. ST toxins are also ADP-ribosylating toxins which activate guanylate cyclase to increase intracellular cGMP. Like cAMP this results in the activation of cyclic nucleotide-dependent protein kinases, protein phosphorylation and opening of the apical membrane chloride channels.

Table II. Bacterial enterotoxins

Enterotoxin	Signal transduction pathways	Accessory pathways
Cholera toxin family		
Cholera toxin	cAMP	5-HT, ENS
E. coli LT-I	cAMP	ENS
E. coli LT-II		
Campylobacter jejuni enterotoxin	cAMP	?
Salmonella enterotoxin	cAMP	?
Shigella enterotoxin (ShET I + II)	cAMP	?
Heat stable toxin family		
E. coli STa	cGMP	ENS
EAST-1	cGMP	?
Y-ST	cGMP	?
NAG-ST	cGMP	?
Other enterotoxins		
Accessory cholera enterotoxin	?	?
Clostridium difficile toxin A	Ca^{++}	cytoskeleton
Enteroinvasive *E. coli* toxin	?	?
Plesiomonas shigelloides LT + ST	?	?
Aeromonas hydrophila enterotoxin	?	?

LT, heat labile toxin; ST, heat stable toxin; EAST-1, enteroaggregative *E. Coli* heat stable toxin 1; Y-ST, *Yersinia enterocolitica* heat stable toxin; NAG-ST, *V. cholera* non-01 heat stable toxin; 5-HT, 5-hydroxytryptamine; ENS, enteric nervous system.

An increasing number of pro-secretory enterotoxins have been discovered during the last few years including accessory cholera toxin (ACE) which increases short circuit current in Ussing chambers, although its precise mode of action has as yet not been clearly defined. Enteroadherent *E. coli* stable toxin (EAST-1) is also a secretory enterotoxin and although known to promote chloride secretion, its effect on intracellular processes within the enterocyte has as yet not been described in detail.

During the past decade it has become evident that bacterial enterotoxins not only interact with the enterocyte promoting chloride secretion and/or inhibiting neutral sodium and chloride absorption, but in many instances act directly or indirectly with other structures within the gut mucosa and submucosa, including inflammatory cells and the enteric nervous system. As stated previously there is increasing evidence that enteric nervous system is involved in the control of intestinal transport processes under basal and other physiological states, and recent evidence indicates that the enteric nervous system is also involved in the pathophysiological disturbances associated with enterotoxin-mediated watery diarrhoea.

Enterotoxins and the enteric nervous system

Neuronal pathways have been implicated in the pertubations of intestinal ion and fluid transport associated with bacterial infection. There is increasing evidence that cholera toxin, *E. coli* enterotoxins, LT and ST and *Clostridium difficile* toxin A produce their secretory effects at least in part *via* a neuronal reflex arc.

Cholera toxin

The first indication that cholera toxin-induced secretion involved the enteric nervous system were *in situ* experiments in cat intestine in which cholera toxin secretion was hibited 60-70% by the neurotoxin, tetrodotoxin, hexamethonium, the nicotinic receptor antagonist, and lignocaine, a local anaesthetic. In these experiments it was not clear however, as to whether cholera toxin activated sub-epithelial neurones or whether the sub-mucosal and/or myenteric plexuses were involved. Involvement in the predominantly cholinergic submucosal plexus is supported by the observation that cholera toxin-induced secretion is inhibited by hexamethonium. Involvement of the mesenteric plexus in cholera toxin secretion was suggested by experiments in Ussing chambers in which "stripped" mucosa, which is largely devoid of the myenteric plexus, was susbtantially impaired in its ability to respond to cholera toxin. In addition, lignocaine was shown to be as effective as tetrodotoxin in inhibiting cholera secretion when applied to the serosal surface of the intestine; localisation studies confirmed that lignocaine had diffused as far as the myenteric plexus and possibly the submucosal plexus but not into the sub-epithelial zone. Chemical ablation studies with benzalkonium chloride which effectively destroys the myenteric plexus, again confirmed its role in cholera secretion. Current evidence suggests therefore that the neuronal reflex involves a sensory afferent type II neurone which is probably cholinergic, an interneurone in the myenteric plexus which has substance

P as the neurotransmitter and a secretory type I neurone which is likely to be VIPergic.

The question remains however, as to how cholera toxin initially activates this reflex pathway. It has been suggested that cholera toxin might directly bind to GM_1 receptors on the sensory afferent nerve in the mucosa. Although there is some evidence to suggest that cholera toxin can penetrate the epithelium, it seems unlikely that sufficient quantities of the holotoxin (84kDa) could target sufficient neuronal tissue to activate the reflex. There is evidence however, that cholera toxin can release a variety of endogenous secretagogues including 5-HT, neurotensin and prostaglandins [5, 13-15].

Cholera toxin has been shown to release 5-HT from enterochromaffin cells; this has been demonstrated by measuring increases in intraluminal 5-HT and depletion of total mucosal 5-HT during cholera secretion. Intraluminal 5-HT concentrations correlate closely with the magnitude of intestinal fluid secretion [16]. Pre-treatment of mammalian intestine *in vivo* with *p*-chlorophenylalanine results in a marked diminution of the intestinal secretory response to cholera toxin. Release of 5-HT is thought to involve an exocytotic process which is calcium-dependent and inhibitable by both L-type and N-type calcium channel blockers. It is proposed that cholera toxin produces enterochromaffin cell degranulation by activation of adenylate cyclase by a similar mechanism to that which occurs in the enterocyte. Cholera toxin induced 5-HT release is modulated by neuronal and humoral factors; muscarinic receptors and β-adrenoreceptors facilitate release where as α_2-adrenoreceptors, histamine, somatostatin, GABA, VIP and PACAP receptors appear to mediate inhibition of release. We have recently shown that 5-HT itself can modulate 5-HT release from entrochromaffin cells *via* 5-HT_3 and 5-HT_4 receptors which are known to exist on enterochromaffin cells [17] ; 5-HT acting *via* 5-HT_3 receptors inhibits further 5-HT release while 5-HT_4 receptors apparently mediate enhancement of release. Thus, autoregulation of enterochromaffin cells by 5-HT is likely to be important both in physiological and pathophysiological states.

5-HT release from enterochromaffin cells is then thought to activate the afferent limb of the neuronal reflex *via* 5-HT_3 and possibly by 5-HT_4 neuronal receptors. The effector limb of the neuronal reflex probably completes the neuronal pathway by releasing VIP which then binds to specific receptors on the basolateral membrane and activates an adenylate cyclase-cAMP intracellular secretory pathway. Interneurones appear to propagate the secretory effects of cholera toxin distally in the small intestine and into the colon. Recent work in mammalian intestine *in situ* indicates that colonic absorption of sodium ions and fluid is reduced by cholera toxin exposure in the proximal small intestine, an effect which is ablated by small intestinal transection; it is presumed that this intervention interferes with the aboral propagation of the secretory neural reflex.

Confirmatory evidence that a 5-HT initiated neural secretory reflex is important in cholera comes from pharmacological inhibition studies in mammalian intestine. Studies in animals have clearly shown that 5-HT_2, 5-HT_3 and 5-HT_4 receptor antagonists can inhibit and in some instances reverse cholera toxin-induced secretion [18-20].

However, the most profound inhibitory effects can only be achieved when the 5-HT antagonist is administered prior to exposure to cholera toxin. Recent studies with the 5-HT_3 receptor antagonist, granisetron suggests that this drug acts predominantly on the enterochromaffin cell [17] itself reducing 5-HT release rather than acting primarily on neuronal 5-HT_3 receptors, thereby blocking the afferent sensory limb of the neural reflex.

Human studies however, have produced conflicting results. The 5-HT_2 receptor antagonist, ketanserin given in combination with the 5-HT_3 receptor antagonist ondansetron, failed to reverse cholera secretion as did the 5-HT_3 receptor antagonist, tropisetron [21]. The 5-HT_3 receptor antagonist, alosetron increased basal sodium and fluid absorption but failed to significantly reduce secretion in a human model of cholera secretion [22]. However, a recent study with the 5-HT_3 receptor antagonist, granisetron reversed fluid and chloride ion secretion to net absorption [23]. The variation in the effects of these 5-HT_3 receptor antagonist may relate to their relative affinities for the 5-HT_3 receptor. ED_{50} of ondansetron, tropisetron and granisetron have been found to be 100, 10 and 5 μg/kg body weight, respectively.

Recent work using substance P antagonists have confirmed a role for this secretagogue and neurotransmitter in cholera toxin secretion. Preliminary studies with the peptide antagonist $DPro^2$-$DTrp^{7,9}SP$ reduced cholera toxin induced secretion but unlike the 5-HT receptor antagonists, failed to convert secretion to absorption [24]. There have been concerns about the specificity of this peptide antagonist and therefore further studies were performed with the non-peptide, highly selective substance P antagonist, CP 96,345 [25]. Again this peptide reduced cholera toxin fluid secretion in a dose-dependent manner, with a parallel reduction in sodium and chloride ion secretion. This agent however, was not able to revert secretion to absorption.

As stated earlier the role of NO in absorptive and secretory processes remains controversial [9, 26]. However, there is some evidence to suggest that nitric oxide may play a role in cholera toxin induced secretion. The nitric oxide synthase inhibitor, L-NAME dose dependently inhibited cholera toxin induced secretion. Interestingly, the NO precursor L-arginine also reduced CT secretion when administered parenterally, although the effect was less marked than with L-NAME [27]. These apparently discordant results may be explained by the proposed dual role for NO in absorptive and secretory processes with actions both on mesenteric blood flow and the enteric nervous system.

The importance of VIP in cholera toxin induced fluid secretion is also supported by inhibition studies [28]. The VIP antagonist, [4Cl-D-Phe_6, Leu_{17}]VIP, converted fluid secretion in rat jejunum to net absorption. Similarly, the sigma receptor agonist, igmesine which reverses VIP-induced increases in short circuit current in mouse ileum mounted in Ussing chambers, reduced cholera toxin induced secretion in rat jejunum *in vivo* and was effective when given both before and following establishment of the secretory state [29].

These observations are entirely consistent with a neural reflex involving 5-HT neural receptors on an afferent sensory neurone, a cholinergic interneurone in the myenteric plexus and a secretory VIPergic, and possibly nitrergic neurone (*figure 2*).

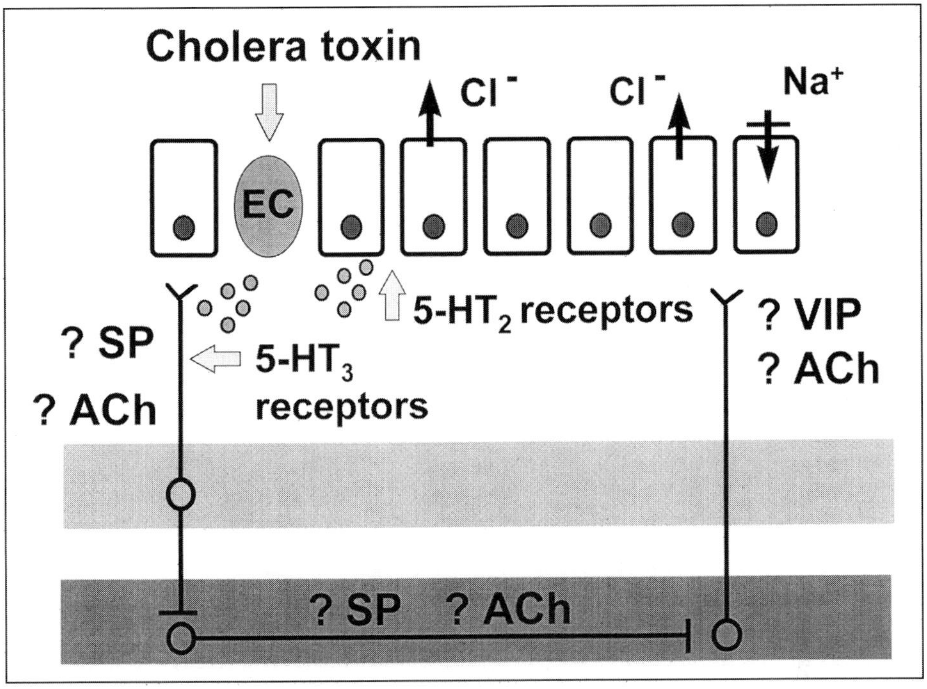

Figure 2. Role of the enteric nervous system in cholera toxin induced intestinal secretion. Current evidence suggests that cholera toxin releases 5-HT from enterochromaffin cells (EC) which acts on 5-HT_2 receptors on enterocytes to promote chloride ion (Cl^-) secretion. In addition, 5-HT is thought to bind neural 5-HT_3 receptors activating a neural reflex involving a substance P/cholinergic interneurone and a VIPergic secretory efferent neurone with activation of VIP receptors on the enterocyte basolateral membrane; this neural reflex results in Cl^- secretion and impaired neutral Na^+ and Cl^- absorption.

E. coli enterotoxins

E. coli LT has marked structural homogeneity with cholera toxin and is known to activate adenylate cyclase in enterocytes. The major difference between the two toxins lies at the cleavage sites between the two components of the A subunit, A_1 and A_2. This results in structural differences between the two toxins at the C terminus of the A_2 chain such that unlike cholera toxin in which A_1 and A_2 subunits have covalently linked, this is not the case with LT. This may account for the observation that LT does not release 5-HT from enterochromaffin cells in the small intestine and that the secretory state induced by this toxin is not inhibitable by 5-HT_2, 5-HT_3 or 5-HT_4 receptor antagonists [20, 30]. Similarly, LT induced secretion is not inhibited by substance P antagonists although the sigma receptor ligand, igmesine does inhibit LT secretion. Despite these differences between cholera toxin and LT, the action of the latter is inhibited by hexamethonium and lignocaine which support the view that the enteric nervous system is involved in LT secretion.

E. coli ST is structurally unrelated to both cholera toxin and LT. The secretory activity of ST does appear to involve the enteric nervous system since fluid secretion is inhibited by tetrodotoxin, lignocaine and hexamethonium [31]. However, like LT, 5-HT release from enterochromaffin cells does not appear to be involved since increased concentrations of 5-HT cannot be detected in the intestinal lumen after ST exposure, nor is there depletion of total mucosal 5-HT. Beubler *et al.* were able to inhibit ST induced fluid secretion using 5-HT_2 and 5-HT_3 receptor antagonists, although we and others have been unable to confirm this observation. NO however, has been implicated in ST induced secretion although neither tetrodotoxin nor the nitric oxide synthase inhibitor, L-NAME affect ST induced changes in short-circuit current in muscle-stripped preparations of pig jejunum and colon. This would support the importance of the myenteric plexus in enterotoxin induced secretory events.

Clostridium difficile toxin A

This cytotoxin is known to produce cell death and necrosis of enterocytes. However, recent studies indicate that neural mechanisms may be involved in the increased intestinal secretion which occurs following exposure to this toxin [32, 33]. Pretreatment of rats with the substance P antagonist CP-96,345 inhibited the increased secretion and increased mannitol permeability in ileal loops exposed to *C. difficile* toxin A. The secretory effects of toxin A were inhibited by lignocaine, hexamethonium and capsaicin indicating the existence of neural patways. In addition, the substance P antagonist also significantly reduced inflammation in the lamina propria and epithelial cell necrosis. It is proposed that cell products from necrotic enterocytes activate primary afferent neurones containing substance P. Substance P is then thought to promote release of secretagogues and chemoattractants from mast cells which produce intestinal secretion and recruit neutrophils which themselves will enhance the secretory process. Substance P released in the vicinity of sub-mucosal arterioles will produce vasodilatation and enhance neutrophil recruitment. Thus, although *Clostridium difficile* toxin A has direct cytotoxic effects on the enterocyte, it would appear that neural reflexes are also involved by enhancing both secretory effects and promoting its role in the pro-inflammatory cascade.

Clinical implications

Although oral rehydration therapy is highly effective in restoring and maintaining fluid and electrolyte balance in enterotoxin-mediated acute watery diarrhoea, the high fluid losses that can occur in cholera are often difficult to keep pace with. Any management intervention which might reduce fluid losses could be of therapeutic benefit. Although it has been known for many years that the ADP-ribosylating toxins activate adenylate and guanylate cyclases there are as yet no therapeutic agents that have been developed to reverse this process. Delineation of accessory mechanisms particularly those involving the enteric nervous system however, do offer therapeutic possibilities since antagonists have already been developed. The demonstration of 5-HT_2, 5-HT_3 and 5-HT_4 receptor antagonists can reverse cholera toxin-induced secretion indicates that this approach may have therapeutic potential. The observation however, that similar effects are not seen with the *E. coli* enterotoxins suggests that this approach may be limited clinically. However, substance P antagonists, VIP antagonists and possibly sigma receptor ligands such as igmesine may have more general applicability in enterotoxin mediated fluid secretion. Further work is clearly needed to establish whether these or related agents will eventually find a place in the treatment of secretory diarrhoea.

References

1. Farthing MJG. Pathophysiology of infective diarrhoea. *Eur J Gastroenterol Hepatol* 1993; 5: 796-807.
2. Goyal RJ, Hirano I. The enteric nervous system. *N Engl J Med* 1996; 334: 1106-15.
3. Furness JB, Bornstein JC. The enteric nervous system and its extrinsic connections. In: Yamada T, ed. *Textbook of Gastroenterology*, 2nd ed. vol 1. Philadelphia: JB Lippincott, 1995; 2-24.
4. Hubel KA. Intestinal nerves and ion transport: stimuli, reflexes and responses. *Am J Physiol* 1985; 248: G261-71.
5. Jodal M. Neuronal influence on intestinal transport. *J Intern Med* 1990; 228: 125-32.
6. Zinner MJ, Jaffe BM, DeMagistis L, Dahlstrom A, Ahlman H. Effect of cervical and thoracic vagal stimulation on luminal serotonin release and regional blood flow in cats. *Gastroenterology* 1982; 82: 1403-8.
7. Ferrara A, Zinner MJ, Jaffe BM. Intraluminal release of serotonin, substance P and gastrin in the canine small intestine. *Dig Dis Sci* 1987; 32: 289-94.
8. Nassar CF, Barada LE, Hamdan AWS, Taha AM, Atewh SF, Saade NE. Involvement of capsaicin-sensitive primary effect fibres in regulation of jejunal alanine absorption. *Am J Physiol* 1995; 268: G695-99.
9. Mourad F, Turvll J, Farthing MJG. The role of nitric oxide in intestinal water and electrolyte transport. *Gut* 1998; in press.
10. MacNaughton WK. Nitric oxide-donating compounds stimulate electrolyte transport in the guinea pig intestine *in vitro*. *Life Sci* 1993; 53: 585-93.
11. Rao RK, Riviere PJ, Pascaud X, Junien JL, Porreca F. Tonic regulation of mouse ileal ion transport by nitric oxide. *J Pharmacol Exp Ther* 1994; 269: 626-31.
12. Maher MM, Gontarek JD, Jimenez RE, Cahill PA, Yeo CJ. Endogenous nitric oxide promotes ileal absorption. *J Surg Res* 1995; 58: 687-92.

13. Cassuto J, Fahrenkrug J, Jodal M, Tuttle R, Lundgren O. Release of vasoactive intestinal polypeptide from the cat small intestine exposed to cholera toxin. *Gut* 1981; 22: 958-63.
14. Munck LK, Mertz-Neilsen A, Westh H, Bukhave K, Beubler E, Rask-Madsen J. Prostaglandin E_2 is a mediator of 5-hydroxytryptamine induced water and electrolyte secretion in the human jejunum. *Gut* 1988; 29: 1337-41.
15. Beubler E, Kollar G, Saria A, Bukhave K, Rask-Madsen J. Involvement of 5-hydroxytryptamine, prostaglandin E_2 and cyclic adenosine monophosphate in cholera toxin-induced fluid secretion in the small intestine of the rat *in vivo*. *Gastroenterology* 1989; 98: 368-76.
16. Bearcroft CP, Perrett D, Farthing MJG. 5-hydroxytrptamine release into human jejunum by cholera toxin. *Gut* 1996; 39: 528-31.
17. Turvill JL, Connor P, Farthing MJG. Enterochromaffin cell 5-HT_3 autoreceptors inhibit cholera toxin (CT)-induced 5-HT release. *Gut* 1997; 41: A39.
18. Beubler E, Horina G. 5-HT_2 and 5-HT_3 receptor subtypes mediate cholera toxin-induced intestinal fluid secretion in the rat. *Gastroenterology* 1990; 99: 83-9.
19. Buchheit KH. Inhibition of cholera toxin-induced intestinal secretion by the 5-HT_3 receptor antagonist ICS 205-930. *Arch Pharmacol* 1989; 339: 704-5.
20. Mourad FH, O'Donnell LJD, Dias JA, Ogutu E, Andre EA, Turvill JL, Farthing MJG. Role of 5-hydroxytryptamine type 3 receptors in rat intestinal fluid and electrolyte secretion induced by cholera and *Escherichia coli* enterotoxins. *Gut* 1995; 37: 340-5.
21. Ehere AJ, Hinterleitner TA, Petritsch W, Holzer Petsche U, Beubler E, Krejs GJ. Effect of 5-hydroxytryptamine antagonists on cholera toxin-induced secretion in the human jejunum. *Eur J Clin Invest* 1994; 24: 664-8.
22. Bearcroft CP, Andre E, Farthing MJG. *In vivo* effects of the 5-HT_3 antagonist alosetron on basal and cholera toxin-induced secretion in the human jejunum: a segmental perfusion. *Aliment Pharmacol Ther* 1997; 11: 1109-14.
23. Turvill JL, Farthing MJG. Effect of granisetron on cholera toxin-induced enteric secretion. *Lancet* 1997; 349: 1293.
24. Turvill JL, Farthing MJG. Substance P (SP) antagonist inhibits cholera toxin but not *E. coli* enterotoxin-induced secretion. *Gastroenterology* 1996; 112: A414.
25. Turvill JL, Connor P, Farthing MJG. Action of non-peptide substance P antagonist, CP 96 345, on cholera toxin and *E. coli* enterotoxin-induced secretion. *Gut* 1998; 42: A25.
26. Mourad FH, O'Donnell LJD, Andre EA, Bearcroft CP, Owen RA, Clark ML, Farthing MJG. L-arginine, nitric oxide and intestinal secretion: studies in rat jejunum *in vivo*. *Gut* 1996; 39: 539-44.
27. Turvill JL, Farthing MJG. Nitric oxide (NO) mediates cholera toxin (CT)-induced secretion in rat small intestine *in vivo*. *Gastroenterology* 1996; 110: A368.
28. Mourad FH, Nassar C. Vasoactive intestinal peptide (VIP) antagonism prevents cholera toxin (CT)-induced fluid secretion in rat jejunum. *Gut* 1997; 41 (Suppl 3): A39.
29. Turvill JL, Kasapidis P, Farthing MJG. Inhibition of cholera toxin (CT)-induced jejunal secretion by the sigma ligand igmesine. *Gastroenterology* 19 ? ?; 112: A414.
30. Turvill JL, Farthing MJG. Selective 5-hydroxytryptamine type 4 (5-HT_4) antagonist inhibits cholera toxin (CT) but not *E. coli* heat labile toxin (LT)-induced secretion. *Gastroenterology* 1996; 110: A368.
31. Eklund S, Jodal M, Lundgren O. The enteric nervous system participates in the secretory response to the heat stable enterotoxins of *Escherichia coli* in rats and cats. *Neuroscience* 1985; 14: 673-81.
32. Pothoulakis H, Castagliuolo I, LaMont T, Jaffer A, O'Keane C, Snider M, Leeman SE. ICP-96,345 a substance P antagonist, inhibits rat intestinal responses to *Clostridium difficile* toxin A but not cholera toxin. *Proc Natl Acad Sci USA* 1994; 91: 947-51.

33. Castagliuolo I, LaMont JT, Letourneau R, Kelly C, O'Keane C, Jaffer A, Theoharides TC, Pothoulakis C. Neuronal involvement in the intestinal effects of *Clostridium difficile* toxin A and *Vibrio* enterotoxin in rat ileum. *Gastroenterology* 1994; 107: 657-65.

Achevé d'imprimer par Corlet, Imprimeur, S.A.
14110 Condé-sur-Noireau (France)
N° d'Imprimeur : 31733 - Dépôt légal : juin 1998
Imprimé en U.E.